Shattering Myths & Mysteries of Alcohol

"A compelling analysis of myths and realities regarding alcohol. Good science. Good teaching. Read and learn. It will help you understand yourself, your family, and your friends. A thoughtful, concise explication of 176 topics related directly to alcohol, its use and abuse. Helpfully presented in alphabetical order."

George D. Lundberg, MD.
Editor-in-Chief, *Journal of the American Medical Association*
American Medical Association
Chicago, Illinois

"An ageless book. I thoroughly enjoyed reading it from cover to cover. The positive messages in it will touch the lives of many readers."

Terry Kelly, Program Director
Drug Free Schools Program
Kamehameha Schools, Community Schools Division
Honolulu, Hawaii

"Dr. Haring's book literally has the power to change lives. The book's greatest strength lies in the way the inspirational messages and scientific findings blend together to make us think twice about our own physical, emotional, and spiritual health. Your book is an absolute winner – no home, school, or library should be without it."

Ava Goldman, Librarian
State of California
Department of Alcohol and Drug Programs

"As I said on the air, I believe your book is one of the best to come out in many years. It is concise and exceptionally user-friendly. It ranks among the top books that I enthusiastically endorse. I continue to recommend it to friends and colleagues."

Neil Scott, Executive Producer
Straight Talk, Recovery Radio for the Northwest
Seattle, Washington

"I just picked up your book and I have not been able to put it down. Not only is it one of the most useful books on alcohol, it is one of the easiest books to follow and understand."

Robert L. Hammond, Executive Director
Alcohol Research Information Service
Lansing, Michigan

"Dr. Haring has produced a treasure-trove of awareness-raisers and denial-busters. A powerful weapon for every councelor's arsenal. I only wish he could have produced the book a decade earlier."

Cliff Creager, CADC, NCAC II
Founding Editor, *Professional Counselor*
Redmond, Washington

"A much needed book. Very well done."

Dan Poynter, Publisher/Author
Para Publishing

"You did it! Your book covers a very personal topic with intelligence and sensitivity. I can only imagine the number of people who will be helped by reading it."

Michael K. Wood, J.D.
California Association of Drinking Driving
TREATMENT Programs (CADDTP)

"A very well written book that clearly spells out the difference between alcohol use, abuse, and dependence. A much needed resource in our school and educational systems."

James Arnold, M.D., Executive Director
California Medical Clinic
San Jose, California

"Shattering Myths & Mysteries of Alcohol appropriately describes this most informative book. Unlike so many in the field of alcoholism, this book deals with, and dispels, the myriad myths that have been around for such a long time. It is great reading not only for those who seek help, but for professionals too."

Jean Kirkpatrick, Ph.D., Founder & Executive Director
Women for Sobriety, Inc.
Quakertown, Pennsylvania

"Dr. Haring's book provokes thought and raises awareness – that is what education for the public aims to do."

Robert G. Kirk, Executive Director
American Council on Alcoholism
Baltimore, Maryland

"Shattering Myths & Mysteries of Alcohol is concise, well organized, and packed with important information written in everyday language. It is encouraging to have current and pertinent information on the impact substance abuse has on individuals, families, and society."

Carolyn Ortiz, Director
Crime and Violence Prevention Center
Department of Justice, State of California

"Your book is fantastic and it is circulating around our office. We have 22 therapists and all are anxious to read your book. Thank you for writing such a worthwhile book."

Sally Thompson, President
New Directions For Youth
Van Nuys, California

"An excellent book for anyone who wants to learn about alcohol. This resource book answers questions about alcohol consumption; surveying myths regarding alcohol and including plenty of practical tips on how to reduce alcohol consumption and strengthen logical decision-making processes."

James A. Cox, Editor-in Chief
The Midwestern Book Review
Oregon, Wisconsin

"Shattering Myths & Mysteries of Alcohol is a well written book that presents straight talk about alcohol and alcohol abuse. The design of the book is clever and the writing style is clear. I can recommend it highly."

Dr. John Preston, Clinical Psychologist, President
Professional School of Psychology
Sacramento, California

"You undoubtedly have a gift for making complex issues understandable. Virtually anyone can pick your book up, read it, and benefit immensely from it. Your book is so valuable I ordered 60 copies to send out to field stations throughout the State of Alabama."

Andrew Milwid, Executive Director
Elks Drug Awareness Program
Dadeville, Alabama

SHATTERING

Myths & Mysteries of Alcohol

Insights & Answers to Drinking, Smoking & Drug Use

by

Raymond V. Haring, Ph.D.

HealthSpan COMMUNICATIONS®

Publisher's Note

This book is solely intended for educational purposes and is not meant whatsoever to serve as a substitute for medical, therapeutic, or any other professional advice or counsel. Assistance involving any aspect of personal health should be addressed by a licensed physician or certified professional in the field.

HealthSpan Communications®
2726 Land Park Drive
Sacramento, California 95818

Visit HealthSpan's Website at: http://www.hspan.com
email: haring@hspan.com
Voice (916) 443-2120 Fax (916) 443-2424

LIBRARY OF CONGRESS
CATALOG CARD NUMBER 97-094070
ISBN 0-9643673-1-9

FOR ADDITIONAL COPIES: CONTACT YOUR BOOKSTORE OR HEALTHSPAN COMMUNICATIONS® (ORDER FORM ON BACK PAGE)

PRINTED IN THE UNITED STATES OF AMERICA

In the middle of every difficulty
lies opportunity.

– Albert Einstein

ACKNOWLEDGMENTS

— To my mother, brother, family, and friends:
All my love.

— To the Stover family:
The dearest friends I will ever have.

— To Paul:
In memory of the gifts you gave.

— To all who have dedicated their lives to helping other people:
Your work will always be remembered and appreciated.

My sincerest appreciation and special thanks are extended
to Gay Carroll and Jackie Boor for their editorial assistance.

Graphic design: Ellen Baxter in association
with HealthSpan Communications.®

Cover photographs: John Klysinski in association
with HealthSpan Communications.®

Cartoons: John Kloss in association with
HealthSpan Communications.®

CONTENTS

PREFACE

Alcohol, or "fermented spirits," has existed since ancient times. Throughout the world, alcohol has played various roles in religious rituals, cultural ceremonies, and social gatherings. From christening ships to toasting newlyweds, it has become woven into the very fabric of our society.

Shattering Myths & Mysteries of Alcohol was written to shed light on numerous issues and concerns regarding alcohol. Presented in alphabetical order for quick and easy reference, this book is a resource guide for anyone seeking information about the dynamics and elements of alcohol and how it affects the mind, body, and soul.

May the words that follow be a means for achieving a better perspective and understanding of alcohol. Alcohol has many faces — the sides that are seen are certain to vary. We may not accept all the statistics, reports, or views of various authorities or agencies — this is to be expected. It is my hope, however, that this book will help dispel many myths and misconceptions regarding alcohol.

Any advice concerning any aspect of one's health should be addressed by a licensed medical doctor or appropriate certified professional in the field.

To your health. Best always,

Raymond V. Haring, Ph.D.

"A thoughtful, concise explication of 176 topics related directly to alcohol, its use and abuse. Helpfully presented in alphabetical order."

— George D. Lundberg, M.D.
Editor-in-Chief, *Journal of the American Medical Association*
American Medical Association

A drink: Just what is a drink? Is it a huge stein of cold beer served at an Old English pub, or perhaps nothing more than a small glass of dessert wine after dinner? As you can see, uncertainty exists as to what constitutes "a drink." The following examples represent the equivalent of a drink, each containing one-half ounce of pure alcohol.

A "Drink"

- 12-ounce beer
- 10-ounce wine cooler
- 3-ounce glass of sherry or port
- 4-ounce glass of (12%) wine
- 1.25 ounces of 80 proof distilled liquor
- 1/2-ounce (12 grams) of pure ethanol

DID YOU KNOW?

Despite drinking less alcohol, women are more vulnerable than men to the effects of alcohol.[1]

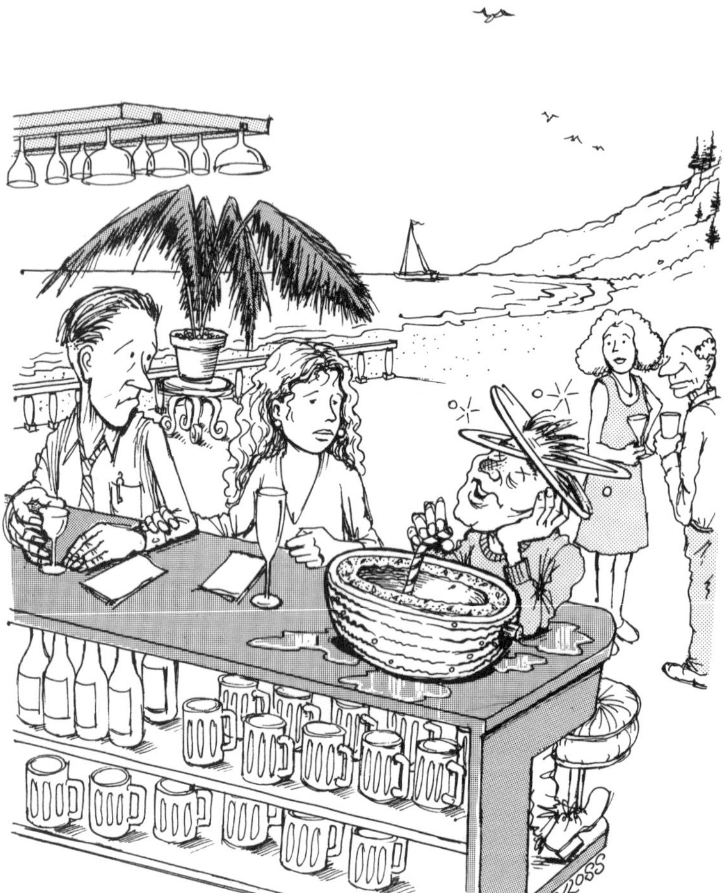

Sometimes – One doesn't equal one!

A quick check for potential alcohol abuse: Is a drinking problem just around the corner? (Refer to section on *abuse of alcohol* for more information.)

Signs of a Drinking Problem

- Feeling uneasy when socializing without a drink
- Being in a hurry to get the first drink
- Finding it difficult to stop drinking after having a drink
- Drinking more as time passes
- Feeling guilty or regretful after drinking
- Looking forward to activities where alcohol is present
- Drinking to ease discomfort of disappointments
- Experiencing memory loss as a result of drinking
- Lying or covering up drinking experiences
- Drinking to reduce stress or responsibilities
- Experiencing the "shakes"
- Planning events that usually lead to heavy drinking
- Losing friends or jobs because of drinking
- Drinking in the morning or early in the day
- Developing relationships with people who drink heavily
- Feeling a need to avoid or curb drinking
- Experiencing behavioral changes when drinking begins

No attempt is made here to diagnose an individual's drinking habits. The more clues or indications, however, that one notices about a person, the more likely there is a problem with alcohol.

A special moment: *A period of time as short as an instant or as long as a lifetime.* Each of us determines how much of our own life is filled with special moments. We are given 1,440 chances, or minutes, each day to find fulfillment and happiness.

The treasures that life holds can elude us if we spend too much time reminiscing about the past or worrying too much about the future. Life is either too short or too long for us to try to alter the past or hurry the future.

> Finish every day and be done with it.
> You have done what you could.
> Some blunders and absurdities no doubt
> crept in; forget them as soon as you can.
>
> Tomorrow is a new day;
> begin it well and serenely
> and with too high a spirit to be cumbered
> with your old nonsense.
>
> This day is all that is good and fair.
> It is too dear, with its hopes and invitations,
> to waste a moment on yesterdays.
>
> —*Ralph Waldo Emerson*

Absorption of alcohol: *The passage of alcohol from the gastrointestinal (GI) tract into the blood system.* The following are two major myths about alcohol absorption:

MYTH

Most alcohol absorption occurs in the stomach.

REALITY

The major site for alcohol absorption is the small intestine, accounting for about 80 percent of all alcohol absorbed into the blood. Less than 25 percent of the alcohol people drink is absorbed in the stomach.

MYTH

Alcohol is absorbed at a fairly steady rate.

REALITY

Many factors can affect the rate of alcohol absorption and, therefore, the rate of alcohol entering the blood. After alcohol enters the blood, it is quickly shipped to the brain. Shortly thereafter, behavioral changes and mood shifts follow the rise in brain alcohol levels.

Alcohol is a powerful disposition-altering drug. After alcohol is absorbed, little can be done to slow down its effect on the body. The type and amount of food present in the stomach significantly affects the rate of alcohol absorption. Foods with a high fat content especially slow the absorption of alcohol.

Bubbles in champagne, sparkling wines and other carbonated alcoholic beverages enhance the effect of a drink. The presence of carbon dioxide speeds up the rate of alcohol.

absorption into the blood.

The rate of alcohol absorption also varies with the types of beverages consumed. The rate of absorption is faster from drinks with higher alcohol content. Drinks loaded with alcohol can put novice drinkers in a tailspin. Drink for drink, heavy drinkers often do not feel the same degree of intoxication from alcohol, because they may have built up a physical tolerance.

DID YOU KNOW?

The activity of stomach enzymes involved in breaking down alcohol is four times greater in men than in women.[2]

The common ulcer drug, cimetidine (Tagamet) decreases the ability of the stomach to burn alcohol. When less alcohol is burned in the stomach, more is headed to the brain and other organs.

Aspirin (acetylsalicylic acid) consumed with alcohol can also enhance blood alcohol levels.

Abstinence: *Voluntary avoidance of all alcohol.* Abstinence means making a conscious decision that drinking will not become a habit or problem. Because alcohol is an addictive drug, for some people, avoiding its use is the only way to ensure that drinking will not become a habit or problem.

MYTH

Heavy drinkers cannot quit drinking.

REALITY

Heavy drinkers are people who drink an average of two or more drinks per day. Many of these drinkers either eventually quit completely or stop drinking for a period of time. The question is not whether a serious drinker can stop, but for how long? The drinker is the only person who can answer this question.

> I've heard him renounce wine a hundred times a day, but then it has been between as many glasses.
>
> — *Douglas Jerrold*

Abuse of alcohol: *In the broadest sense, alcohol abuse refers to any misuse of alcohol.* Surely drunkenness and alcoholism reflect abuse; however, alcohol abuse occurs whenever an individual consumes enough alcohol to cause any kind of problem.

For example, consider a woman who occasionally drinks light to moderate amounts of alcohol during pregnancy. Even though she may consider herself a light social drinker, she is abusing alcohol. No alcohol is recommended for women during pregnancy.

To eliminate any uncertainty of a clinical diagnosis of alcohol abuse, the American Psychiatric Association's current *Diagnostic and Statistical Manual (DSM-IV)* lists various criteria that must be met:

Is a Person Abusing Alcohol?

The American Psychiatric Association's Diagnostic and Statistical Manual *DSM-IV* outlines symptoms used to diagnose substance (alcohol) abuse.

Group A response:

A pattern of alcohol use resulting in "clinically significant impairment or distress," as exhibited by one or more of the following conditions within a 12-month period:

- ☐ Repeated use of alcohol that results in the failure to fulfill major obligations.
- ☐ Use of alcohol in situations when it is physically hazardous.
- ☐ Recurrent alcohol-related legal problems (e.g., breaking the law by disorderly conduct).
- ☐ Continued use of alcohol in spite of repeated social or interpersonal problems triggered or made worse by alcohol use.

Group B response:

- ☐ The person's symptoms have not met the criteria for Alcohol Dependence. (See section on alcohol dependence.)

A diagnosis for alcohol abuse occurs when at least one positive response in section A and a positive response in section B is met. The severity of alcohol abuse is a function of the number of positive symptoms and the severity of those symptoms.

Adapted and reprinted with permission from the Diagnostic and Statistical Manual of Mental Disorders, Fourth Edition. Copyright 1994 American Psychiatric Association.

MYTH

Alcohol abusers will eventually become alcoholics.

REALITY

The odds are stacked against anyone who abuses alcohol over a period of time. If people drink to relax and have fun, escape from responsibilities and pressures, loosen up to feel more sociable and accepted, or drink just to ease the discomfort of low self-esteem, they are at a higher risk of abusing alcohol than people who drink infrequently.

Any time alcohol is used as a means of escaping to feel better about life, a habit is in the making. Each drink fuels the fire for alcohol abuse and the potential for developing a dependency.

Personal alcohol use could be viewed metaphorically as a circle, starting with the first drink and continuing all the way around to the last drink of one's life. People who rarely use alcohol spend very little time navigating the circle.

Heavy drinkers spend more time on the "drinking wheel." For them, each cycle of drinking ends the way it begins, a step closer to their destiny, but with no greater vision of the end in sight. It is no great mystery that the more one drinks, the less time and energy a person has to pursue other interests.

People Should Not Drink if They:

- Want to eliminate any chance of developing alcohol dependence
- Are pregnant (or attempting to conceive) or lactating
- Experience circulatory problems such as:
    - – coronary artery disease
    - – congestive heart failure
    - – hypertension
- Suffer from other medical disorders such as:
    - – gastrointestinal ulcers
    - – gout
    - – diabetes
    - – depression or anxiety
- Drive or operate heavy equipment
- Take drugs or medications that interact with alcohol
- Have a predisposition to developing alcohol dependence
- Are under the age of 21

Note: This list represents only a small sample of conditions that reflect the need to avoid alcohol. When in doubt, it is advisable to consult a health care professional who can provide you with a useful resource.

Achievement: *Accomplishment of a goal.* Whether a goal is to improve health, abstain from alcohol, reduce stress or become more physically fit, achievement comes one step at a time.

To achieve any goal, people must set their sights on something they want and then visualize it in detail. The goal will then become a "target" upon which to aim.

Do you have a particular goal that you would like to accomplish? If so, write it down on a piece of paper. Congratulations! You have done the hardest work so far. The next step is to take small measured steps toward that goal each day. Anything ever built, learned or changed, happened one step at a time.

> The heights by great men reached and kept
> were not attained by sudden flight,
> but they, while their companions slept,
> were toiling upward in the night.
>
> — *Henry Wadsworth Longfellow*

Regardless of size, any step toward meeting a goal is an action step. Good intentions are not sufficient to get the job done. The most well-developed plan has little value, unless action supports its design.

> Are you in earnest? Seize this very minute —
> What you can do, or dream you can, begin it,
> Boldness has genius, power, and magic in it.
> Only engage, and then the mind grows heated —
> Begin it, and the work will be completed!
>
> — *Goethe*

Start this minute. Identify one goal. Estimate the completion date. Write down the actions you will take to complete your goal. Use the following table as a guide:

Sample Action Steps

Goal: Exactly what do you want? Be specific.

Immediately relieve tension without drinking.

How long will it take?

30 to 40 minutes!

What needs to happen?

Lie on the floor. Stretch for four to five minutes. Breathe deeply from diaphragm. Play with the dog for a few minutes before taking a brisk walk through the park. Build a nice fire after dinner.

Action Steps

Goal: Exactly what do you want? Be specific.

How long will it take?

What needs to happen?

Acute: *Something that develops suddenly and usually lasts a short time. Acute* drinking generally refers to a single episode of drinking. In contrast, *chronic* drinking refers to the prolonged use of alcohol.

MYTH

Long-term drinking is always more dangerous than short-term drinking.

REALITY

A single episode of drinking can have lasting harmful effects and even be life threatening. Consider the New Year's Eve celebrant who ties on a good one just once a year and ends up contributing to the tragic number of highway accidents and fatalities. Or consider the pregnant woman who decides to drown her discomfort in what she mistakenly thinks is a safe amount of alcohol. She directly risks the future health of her unborn child.

Addiction: *An overwhelming habit, compulsion or craving.* Regardless of the definition, addiction implies a physical dependence on a drug. Once a physical dependence has developed, drug use must be maintained in order to prevent physical withdrawal. (Refer to section on *alcohol dependence.*)

DID YOU KNOW?

Naltrexone has been approved by the FDA to be used in the treatment of alcoholism.

MYTH

"Hard liquor" is required to develop an alcohol addiction.

REALITY

Interestingly, many people do not realize alcohol in any beverage is a potential problem. Alcohol is an addicting drug, regardless if it is wine, beer, champagne or distilled spirits such as vodka, gin, bourbon or whiskey. In general, it is the amount of alcohol and the length of time one drinks that determines the risk of developing an addiction.

Adipose tissue: *The body fat we wear from consuming too many calories.*

MYTH

Alcohol cannot be converted to body fat.

REALITY

Alcohol is rich in calories (7 calories/gram) and has a tremendous impact on the liver's ability to make fat. Lipogenesis is the fancy term for making fat. When alcohol is broken down in the liver, powerful biochemical instructions are given to the liver to increase fat synthesis. The liver listens very carefully. Once fat is made in the liver, it is shipped out to be used or stored in adipose tissue. A flabby, soft body can result from excessive drinking and eating.

Fat, also known as triglycerides, is sometimes confused with adipose tissue. This specialized tissue actually stores the fat we produce as a result of consuming more calories than we need to meet our energy needs.

Typically, a pound of body fat is stored somewhere in the body for every 3,500 calories we overeat or drink. One ounce of alcohol supplies a whopping 210 calories, the equivalent of six teaspoons of lard. Do not be fooled. Even though alcohol may be clear as water, it looks very different on our bodies.

Adversity: *A hardship or grief suffered and endured.* You are not alone if you have ever experienced a difficult situation. Tens of millions of people around the world experience pain associated with alcohol abuse.

Living as a victim helps no one. Tossing the victim role and reaching for something positive turns adversity to one's favor. All people are dealt a deck of cards in life. How they play the card game can change their perspective and have an enormous effect on their attitude.

Rather than thinking of adversities as problems, think of them as challenges. Overcoming challenges bolsters self-esteem. Treating challenges as misfortunes erodes the spirit and soon becomes counterproductive.

It may seem simplistic to change an attitude by merely changing the words that describe a situation, but it works. Life can become overwhelming if we make things larger than they are by using inappropriate words.

Growth occurs when nurtured by resistance. We are all faced with challenges. Regardless of the hurdles that may face us, we can find comfort in knowing that joy and pleasure are the rewards of overcoming adversities.

> A man of character finds a special attractiveness in difficulty, since it is only by coming to grips with difficulty that he can realize his potentialities.
>
> — *Charles de Gaulle*

The Use of Words Can Change Thoughts

SAY YES	Change is easier than I think.
NEVER	It will take me forever to change.
SAY YES	I will meet some very nice people.
NEVER	I drink because I hate being alone.
SAY YES	I will enjoy my life without drinking.
NEVER	I can't relax without a drink.
SAY YES	I find happiness without drinking.
NEVER	Drinking is delightful.
SAY YES	I will succeed.
NEVER	I'm never going to make it.
SAY YES	I will do things that make me relaxed.
NEVER	I'm always stressed.
SAY YES	Life is wonderful.
NEVER	Life is tough and then you die.
SAY YES	I will stop drinking.
NEVER	I can't control my drinking.
SAY YES	I will be in the best shape of my life.
NEVER	I'll always be out of shape.

Be careful what you tell yourself. People who tell themselves they can't stop drinking find it almost unbearable to quit. Throughout history, people have shaped their future by endorsing a positive attitude.

Affirmations: *Positive phrases, concepts or images rehearsed over and over in one's mind.* Making affirmations is a way of gently preparing the mind to accept new ways of thinking and doing things.

By sending positive signals to the brain, affirmations can be a powerful tool for drinkers who want to change their drinking habits. Nothing seems to be more inspiring and bolstering to your attitude than affirmations that abound with enthusiasm and optimism.

Have you ever gotten tired of pleasant soothing thoughts, comforting suggestions or a bandwagon full of cheering supporters? Sometimes it only takes a glimmer of cheer or hope to change our entire view of the world. That smidgen of faith may be found in as little as two words: I can.

> They are able
> because they think they are able.
>
> — *Vergil*

Some people find encouragement from the compliments paid by friends or peers. Still others find affirmations attached to a refrigerator door more invigorating than drinking a full pot of brewed coffee in the morning.

The practice of positive affirmations has been used for years by people from all walks of life. Sports enthusiasts, psychotherapists, health trainers and countless health care professionals recognize the value of practicing positive affirmations. Although affirmations are not cure-alls, they offer a way of sending positive, uplifting signals to the brain; there are, however, a few limitations to their use.

For example, no one would say, "Gee whiz, my house just burned down, and I broke my leg. Isn't life wonderful!"

As this outlandish example shows, the point of an affirmation is not to mislead or indicate that everything is okay. Rather, affirmations should offer direction and guidance, producing an inner sense of well-being that allows people to accept a new belief.

Consider a person who believes it is very difficult, if not impossible, to stop drinking. Imagine a negative affirmation on the refrigerator door that reads, "I have no control and never will have any control over my drinking habits." That person would eventually start to believe that he or she has no control. On the other hand, positive affirmations, such as, "I am in control. I am responsible for my choices. I can change my drinking habits" can be a tremendous support system.

It is not enough to just rehearse positive affirmations in one's mind. To make affirmations more beneficial, the following suggestions should prove helpful:

Affirmations

It feels great to be drug-free.
It feels great to be drug-free.
It feels great to be drug-free.

It is wonderful to feel healthy.
It is wonderful to feel healthy.
It is wonderful to feel healthy.

Suggestions

- Be as relaxed as possible. It is impossible to grasp an affirmation in a rushed, agitated, or anxious state.
- Challenge the old belief. It is easier to substitute a new belief if the old belief seems unrealistic.
- Employ a sense of certainty when developing an affirmation. Avoid language like, "Maybe." Instead, use words such as "I can."
- The affirmation should be realistic. Unobtainable affirmations are not believable.
- Visualize in detail the benefits of the affirmation.
- Write down your affirmation in present tense.

Al-Anon: *An auxiliary organization of Alcoholics Anonymous founded in the mid-1950s to lend support to family members of alcoholics.* Members learn how to live without contributing to or magnifying problems in the alcoholic-family unit.

Al-Anon members are encouraged to adopt AA's Twelve-Step Program as a foundation for developing a supportive life-style. They learn that they are powerless over the alcoholic's drinking problem. Although Al-Anon is run by lay people, it is considered a positive source of guidance for family members struggling with alcohol abusers.

Alateen: *An auxiliary organization of Alcoholics Anonymous that addresses problems of teenagers living with alcoholic parents.* Alateen grew out of the tremendous success of Al-Anon.

DID YOU KNOW?

All states have established that 21 years of age is the legal age for drinking alcoholic beverages.

Alcohol: *A colorless, chemical liquid clinically known as ethanol or ethyl alcohol.* Sometimes called grain alcohol, alcohol is produced from the fermentation of carbohydrates. It is the intoxicating substance present in beverages such as beer, wine and distilled or "hard" liquor such as bourbon, rum, vodka, brandy, and whisky.

At a glance, it is difficult to appreciate that such a tiny, simple compound born out of sugar could wield such an enormous effect on humans. While alcohol consumption produces a variety of biochemical, physiological, and psychological effects, it can also have a profound effect on friendships, families, and careers. In 1990 alone, the effects of alcohol cost our society over 100 billion dollars in loss of life, injuries, sickness, and loss of productivity.

DID YOU KNOW?

Although 70 percent of the American population drink alcohol, approximately one-half of all alcohol is consumed by 10 percent of the drinkers.[3]

Alcohol dehydrogenase (ADH): Although burdensome to pronounce, and generally mentioned only in medical schools or biochemistry laboratories, these particular enzymes are critical to sobering a person after a bout with drinking.

Have you ever wondered how the body actually battles

with alcohol? It is fairly simple. Tiny specialized proteins, called enzymes, start dismantling alcohol the instant the enzymes and alcohol come into contact. Typically, the battalion of alcohol fighters, which biochemists call alcohol dehydrogenase enzymes, are located in the liver.

With heavy or prolonged drinking bouts, additional enzyme recruits are called in to help wrestle the excess alcohol out of the body. Aside from its unattractive and rather long name, the microsomal ethanol-oxidizing system, or MEOS system, should receive a merit badge for its assistance in ridding the body of excess alcohol.

Since other drugs can use the same MEOS alcohol burning system, potential drug interaction may exist when two or more drugs are taken at the same time.

Mixing alcohol and other drugs can be extremely dangerous. If two or more drugs are vying for the same oxidizing system, a time delay may be experienced in the degradation of either drug. This could cause one or more of the drugs to linger in the blood longer, synergistically increasing that particular drug's effect.

With certain drugs, this could prove disastrous. With thousands of drugs on the market, it is no wonder it makes good sense to check with your doctor or pharmacist about potential drug interactions.

DID YOU KNOW?

Although light use of alcohol can interfere with the breakdown of certain drugs such as barbiturates, diazepam (tranquilizing drugs), and phenytoin (antiseizure drugs), heavy alcohol use can increase their degradation rate.[4]

Alcohol dependence: *Characterized by tolerance to alcohol and physical withdrawal symptoms when a person abstains from alcohol consumption.* In simple terms, the person has a serious problem with alcohol.

It is no mystery that some people can drink larger amounts of alcohol with less noticeable effects. This phenomenon is called *tolerance*. Habitual use of a drug increases tolerance to it. Either the liver becomes more effective in handling the drug, or the body tissues become less sensitive to the drug.

Stages of alcohol dependence

Virtually by imperceptible transition, alcohol dependence can develop over time. Traditionally, four stages of alcohol dependence are recognized:

Stage One: A person can tolerate more alcohol consumption without noticing deleterious effects; they can function and perform normally.

Stage Two: The person cannot recall certain events that occurred during episodes of drinking.

Stage Three: A person's control over drinking is lost. The person becomes more dependent on alcohol with continued drinking. Withdrawal symptoms, which entail an intense craving or irresistible urge for a drink, are evident if the person stops drinking.

Stage Four: The person exhibits a sustained or prolonged pattern of drunkenness. Significant loss and deterioration of vital physiological processes are likely.

DID YOU KNOW?

Rates of alcohol abuse and dependency are higher among males than among females.[5]

There are varying degrees of dependence, tolerance, and withdrawal symptoms associated with excessive drinking. The American Psychiatric Association's current *Diagnostic and Statistical Manual (DSM-IV)* distinguishes between alcohol abuse and alcohol dependence. The following table describes the criteria used to diagnose alcohol dependence:

Who is Dependent on Alcohol?

The American Psychiatric Association's Diagnostic and Statistical Manual *DSM-IV* outlines symptoms used to diagnose Alcohol Dependence.

A pattern of alcohol use resulting in "clinically significant impairment or distress," as exhibited by three or more of the following conditions at any time within a 12-month period:

- ☐ **Alcohol tolerance,** as determined by either of the following criteria:
  – a need to drink significantly more alcohol to "achieve intoxication or a desired effect."
  – a substantially reduced effect with continued use of comparable amounts of alcohol.
- ☐ **Alcohol withdrawal,** as determined by the "Diagnostic Criteria for Alcohol Withdrawal." The guidelines are listed in the withdrawal section of this book.
- ☐ Alcohol is consumed in larger amounts or over a longer time period than the person intended.
- ☐ A persistent desire or unsuccessful attempts to control or reduce alcohol use.
- ☐ Considerable time spent to obtain, use or recover from the effects of alcohol.
- ☐ Social, occupational or recreational activities have been missed or reduced because of alcohol use.
- ☐ Continued use of alcohol despite knowing that physical, psychological or social problems are exacerbated by its use.

Note: A diagnosis for alcohol dependence occurs when at least three positive responses are met within the same 12-month period. Physical dependence is present when either alcohol tolerance or withdrawal is present.

Adapted and reprinted with permission from the Diagnostic and Statistical Manual of Mental Disorders, Fourth Edition. Copyright 1994 American Psychiatric Association.

Alcohol in medications: It is incredibly easy to stay informed about the alcohol content in medications. Manufacturers of products containing alcohol must disclose the information on product labels. Many equally effective, nonalcoholic substitutes are on the market.

Unless specifically advised by a physician, recovering alcoholics should be particularly careful to avoid various cold, cough, and congestion preparations containing alcohol. Their physicians should be aware that they are recovering alcoholics with a history of alcohol abuse.

Consulting a pharmacist or physician eliminates doubt about the alcohol content of a particular medication. The following tables mention only a small fraction of drugs and medications that contain alcohol.

DID YOU KNOW?

More than 100 medications have potentially harmful drug interactions with alcohol, especially drugs such as anticonvulsants, antidepressants, antianxiety, sedative, sleeping pills that depress the brain, and certain pain relievers.[6]

Drugs Containing Alcohol Used for Cold, Cough, Congestion, and Allergy

Drug	Alcohol proof
Actifed w/ Codeine (Rx)	8.6
Benylin Cough	10
Dimetane	6
Dimetane - DC (RX)	1.9
Duratuss - HD (RX)	10
Hycotuss (RX)	20
Novahistine Expectorant (RX)	15
Novahistine DI I (RX)	15
Nucofed Expectorant	24
Nucofed Ped Expectorant	12
NyQuil Cold & Flu	20
Pediacof (RX)	10
Periactin Syrup (RX)	10
Phenergan Syrup Plain (RX)	14
Promethazine (DM, VC, C) (RX)	14
Robitussin AC (RX)	7
Vicks Formula 44E Cough & Chest	20
Vicks Formula 44M	20

This table represents only a small list of drugs reported to contain alcohol. Product content may change. Always refer to literature accompanying product for certainty of alcohol content. Percent alcohol is one-half alcohol proof. (RX) designates a prescription drug. The intent of this table is only to create an awareness that certain drugs may contain alcohol.

Alcohol-free Drugs Used for Cold, Cough, Congestion, Allergy

Actifed Syrup
Benadryl Elixir*
Childrens' Nyquil Cold/Cough
Childrens' Tylenol Cold
Deconamine Syrup (RX)
Delsym Cough
Dimetapp Elixir
Histussin HC
Hycodan (RX)
Hycomine (RX)
Naldecon Syrup (RX)
Naldecon Ped Syrup (RX)
Nucofed Syrup* (RX)
Polyhistine - DM (RX)
Polyhistine - CS (RX)
Ryna C Liquid (RX)
Sudafed Child liquid
Triaminic Syrup
Triaminicol
Tussiorganidin - DM (RX)
Tussiorganidin - C (RX)
Tussionex (RX)

This table does not represent a complete list of drugs reported to be "alcohol-free." Product content may change. Always refer to literature accompanying product for certainty of content. (RX) designates a prescription drug. *Note: Certain brands of Benadryl Elixir may contain alcohol. Nucofed *Ped Expectorant* and Nucofed *Expectorant* contain alcohol. Carefully check manufacturer's label. The intent of this table is only to create an awareness that certain drugs may be alcohol-free.

Various Alcohol-free Drugs

Analgesics

Acetaminophen Plain Liquid* (RX)
Demerol Syrup (RX)

Antiasthmatic

Elixophyllin -GG Liquid (RX)
Slo-Phyllin Syrup (RX)

Anticonvulsants

Mysoline Suspension (RX)
Tridione Suspension (RX)

Antidiarrheals

Kaopectate Suspension
Pepto-Bismol

Antipsychotics

Haldol Concentrate (RX)
Stelazine Concentrate (RX)
Thorazine Syrup (RX)
Thorazine Concentrate (RX)

This table does not represent a complete list of drugs reported to be "alcohol-free." Always refer to literature accompanying product for certainty of content. Product content may change. (RX) designates a prescription drug. *Note: Certain brands may contain alcohol. The intent of this table is only to create an awareness that certain drugs may be alcohol-free. Carefully check manufacturer's label.

Common Drugs Containing Alcohol

Drug	Alcohol proof
Acetaminophen + Codeine (RX)	15
Benadryl Elixir*	28
Donnagel	8
Donnatal Elixir (RX)	46
Dramamine Liquid	10
Entex (RX)	10
Feosol	10
Elixophyllin (RX)	40
Gevrabon	36
Ipecac Syrup	4
Lanoxin Elixir Ped. (RX)	20
Lortab (RX)	14
Organidine (RX)	43
Phenobarbital (RX)	27
Tagamet liquid (RX)	6

This table represents only a small list of drugs reported to contain alcohol. Always refer to literature accompanying product for certainty of alcohol content. Product content may change. Percent alcohol is one-half alcohol proof. (RX) designates a prescription drug. *Note: Certain brands of Benadryl Elixir may not contain alcohol. Carefully check manufacturer's label. The intent of this table is only to create an awareness that certain drugs may contain alcohol.

Alcohol intoxication: *A drug-altered condition that affects mental and physical functioning.* Measuring the percentage of alcohol in the blood (blood alcohol concentration, or "BAC") is useful in determining the degree of intoxication.

For some people, the slightest amount of alcohol seems to be sufficient to qualify for intoxication. Obviously, varying degrees exist.

Typically, the effect of alcohol on the body begins with the first drink. It may actually remove inhibitions and relax the person. In some people, this feeling may trigger a desire for another drink.

So, what about the second drink, the third drink and more? The truth is, with each drink the brain becomes more impaired.

DID YOU KNOW?

Federal regulations prohibit pilots from flying an aircraft within eight hours of consuming any beverage containing alcohol, or if pilots have blood alcohol levels of 0.04 percent or higher.[7]

Alcohol's Effect on Brain Function

Level of Intoxication (% Blood Alcohol Level)	
0.02 – 0.05	impaired judgment • euphoric mood mind & body at ease • relaxed
0.08 – 0.10	• legally intoxicated • impaired coordination • delayed reaction time
0.15	impaired vision • slurred speech seriously impaired judgment
0.2	inability to walk without help
0.3 – 0.4	stuporous • out-of-control inability to understand
0.4 – 0.7	unconsciousness • coma • death

DID YOU KNOW?

> It is the quantity of alcohol consumed, not the act of mixing alcoholic drinks, that leads to intoxication.

The American Psychiatric Association's current *Diagnostic and Statistical Manual (DSM-IV)* outlines the criteria used to diagnose alcohol intoxication:

Diagnostic Criteria for Alcohol Intoxication

The American Psychiatric Association's Diagnostic and Statistical Manual *DSM-IV* outlines criteria used to diagnose Alcohol Intoxication.

Group A response:

- ☐ Recent consumption of alcohol.

Group B response:

- ☐ Clinically significant behavioral or psychological changes that result during or shortly after alcohol has been ingested.

  – inappropriate or aggressive behavior
  – inappropriate sexual conduct
  – impaired judgment, etc.

Group C response:

- ☐ One or more of the following manifestations result during or shortly after alcohol has been ingested:

  – coma or stupor
  – impaired memory or attention
  – incoordination
  – nystagmus (involuntary eye movement)
  – slurred speech
  – unsteady gait (walking or stepping)

Group D response:

- ☐ The symptoms above are not a result of an existing medical condition or another mental disorder.

Note: Criteria A-D are essential features of alcohol intoxication. The degree of alcohol intoxication is related to the severity of symptoms.

Alcohol metabolism: There is enough written on this subject to fill a football stadium. Let's keep it simple. First, use "little changes" to replace the word metabolism. Metabolism can be a daunting word. Simply put, it means something will either be broken down to smaller pieces, or little pieces will be hooked together to make something larger.

Alcohol is unusual in that it can be either metabolized as a source of energy or chemically changed to be stored as body fat. In other words, the body does not have a storage site for alcohol. Any alcohol consumed will continue to circulate in the body until it is metabolized.

Men metabolize alcohol differently than women. In men, about a quarter of the alcohol consumed can be burned in the gastrointestinal tract (GI tract). This means that less alcohol is actually absorbed into their bloodstream to be carried to the brain. In women, more alcohol is absorbed by the body because their GI tract metabolizes less alcohol than does a man.

In both men and women, a very small amount of alcohol (about five percent) can be exhaled by breathing. This is the basis for the use of breathalyzers that detect alcohol on a person's breath.

MYTH

Walking or running helps a person to sober up.

REALITY

This is wishful thinking for those people who have had too much to drink. Muscles can burn sugars and fats, but they have no machinery to burn alcohol. Although the stomach can burn significant quantities of alcohol, especially in men, the liver is the major site where alcohol is burned.

Many people imagine that if they walk or run after they drink, that the physical exercise will help burn alcohol. Time, however, is the real catalyst. More to the point, the liver needs time to eliminate alcohol from the body. Alcohol is burned at an almost constant rate, regardless of what we do.

DID YOU KNOW?

How Fast are Alcoholic Drinks Burned?

Rates of alcohol metabolism vary to some extent from person to person. Most people burn between **0.25** to **0.50** ounces of pure alcohol per hour.

One-half ounce of pure alcohol is considered one drink. The following drinks contain approximately 0.5 ounces of pure alcohol:

- 12-ounce beer
- 10-ounce wine cooler
- 3-ounce glass of sherry or port
- 4-ounce glass of (12%) wine
- 1.25 ounces of 80 proof distilled liquor
- 1/2-ounce (12 grams) of pure ethanol

Alcohol-related disorders: *Afflictions and ailments caused by drinking alcohol.*

MYTH

The toxic effects of alcohol are limited to liver and brain damage.

REALITY

The path of destruction caused by excessive drinking extends far beyond the brain and liver. The disruption of many bodily functions is just the beginning. Permanent impairment and loss of life can be the more serious consequences of alcohol abuse. The list below mentions some common alcohol-related disorders:

- Cancer of esophagus, larynx, stomach, liver and colon
- Hypertension, stroke and heart disease
- Damage to the pancreas, kidneys and brain
- Gastrointestinal (GI) ulcers
- Birth defects
- Impotence and infertility
- Diminished immunity
- Increased susceptibility to infections and diseases
- Sleep disturbances
- Impaired physical and mental performance

Alcoholic: *A person who is physically dependent on alcohol.* In 1980, the American Psychiatric Association substituted *alcohol dependence syndrome* for the term *alcoholism.* (For more information, refer to sections on *alcoholism* and *alcohol dependence.*)

Alcoholic liver disease: *Any illness or damage to the liver caused by alcohol ingestion.* The extent of liver damage is usually related to the duration and quantity of alcohol consumed.

Fatty liver is the most common liver disease among people who abuse alcohol. Alcoholic hepatitis, a more severe form of liver disease, is characterized by inflammation of the liver. The most severe form of liver disease, cirrhosis, is an irreversible disease characterized by extensive scarring of the liver.

Alcoholics Anonymous (AA): *An organization founded in 1935 by Bill Wilson and Bob Smith, both recovered alcoholics.* AA is a worldwide organization made up of local chapters offering regular group meetings that help fellow recovering alcoholics maintain sobriety. The basic principles of Alcoholics Anonymous are reflected in its Twelve-Step Program. Basic tenets of AA's philosophy are as follows:

Alcoholics Anonymous is not a religious organization. Although God is mentioned in their program, members are free to follow their own faith and religious beliefs.

AA is effective because it provides a forum for fellow members to offer understanding, compassion and emotional support for maintaining sobriety and building a satisfying life free of alcohol. There is no substitute for attending an AA meeting. The warmth and encouragement provided by its members create an invaluable support system. (For more information, refer to section on AA's *Twelve-Step Program.*)

Alcoholism: *Alcohol dependence, often referred to as alcoholism, is a disease characterized by physical dependence on alcohol and an impaired ability to control its consumption.*

In the home or on the streets, alcoholism describes an existence that is bound and shackled to a bottle of alcohol. Defining alcoholism has been a tough problem. Satisfying all authorities in the field would be like counting stars or defining love. It is a difficult task.

Alcoholism is characterized by the compulsive and excessive consumption of alcohol to the point that an individual develops tolerance and physical dependence on alcohol. (Refer to section on *alcohol dependence*, which discusses the American Psychiatric Association's current guidelines for alcohol dependence.)

> "Alcoholism is a primary, chronic disease with genetic, psychosocial and environmental factors influencing its development and manifestations. The disease is often progressive and fatal. It is characterized by continuous or periodic impaired control over drinking, preoccupation with the drug alcohol, use of alcohol despite adverse consequences, and distortions in thinking, most notably denial."
>
> *— National Council on Alcoholism and Drug Dependence, Inc. and the American Society of Addiction Medicine.*

MYTH

A majority of drinkers will eventually become alcoholics.

REALITY

It is difficult to gauge exactly how many people in the United States are alcohol-dependent drinkers. Regardless of the number, millions of people who are alcoholics are found in all sectors of society, including young and old, male and female, affluent and poor. Although it is generally accepted that alcoholism cannot be cured, it can be diagnosed and treated. Studies show that at least one in 10 drinkers will become an alcoholic.

MYTH

Its chemical nature is the only reason people become addicted to alcohol.

REALITY

There is no single cause or reason that leads a person to alcoholism. Alcoholism is not a disease one "catches" like a cold or flu. The disease develops through repeated use of alcohol over a period of time. A person is unlikely to become an alcoholic without continuous exposure to alcohol. An individual's history of alcohol use can determine the likelihood of becoming an alcoholic.

Although alcohol is the agent of alcoholism, it cannot be considered the only explanation as to why people drink until a physical dependence develops. If alcohol were the sole factor, then people taking their first drink would conceivably continue until addiction occurred. The susceptibility to alcoholism is influenced by five factors. All are thought to contribute in some way to the development of a drinking problem:

- Addictive nature of alcohol
- Personality traits
- Genetic factors
- Environmental factors
- Lack of knowledge

Millions of people drink on occasion. When drinking becomes routine, people position themselves on a track that can lead to alcohol dependency.

Heavy drinkers who consume several drinks a day on a continuing basis are more likely to abuse alcohol and become alcohol dependent. When people feel physically or emotionally uncomfortable without a drink, control over their drinking may be in doubt. Health, family and work problems significantly related to alcohol can occur well before a person has developed alcohol dependence.

Amnesia: *Diminished ability to recall information from memory.*

DID YOU KNOW?

Temporary memory loss from drinking is a warning sign of alcoholism. Whether or not a person is an alcoholic, excessive drinking can result in both short and long-term memory impairment.

Analgesic: *A drug with painkilling properties.*

DID YOU KNOW?

> Alcohol is a poor analgesic because of the quantity required to effectively relieve pain.

Anemia: *A condition characterized by a deficiency in red blood cells (RBCs), or in the amount of hemoglobin (oxygen carrying pigment in RBCs) they contain.* Like most cells in the body, red blood cells wear out and need to be replenished on a regular basis.

Due to the enormous number of RBCs that need replacement every day, it is important to have the essential nutrients to manufacture and nourish them.

An iron deficiency caused by poor eating habits is just one cause of anemia. A deficiency of vitamin B12 and folic acid, both commonly found to be low in drinkers, can lead to *pernicious* and *megaloblastic* anemia, respectively. The result is similar. The capacity to carry oxygen by these large, defective red blood cells is significantly impaired.

MYTH

Wine is a good source of iron and other nutrients.

REALITY

Wine is a very poor source of iron. An adult woman would have to consume 35 glasses of red wine to meet her daily recommendation for iron. A man would need to drink 20 glasses of red wine to meet his daily recommendation.

The same holds true for other nutrients. Alcoholic drinks have little, if any, nutritional value. (Refer to the table in the section, *nutritional value of alcoholic beverages.*) Major nutritional deficiencies and medical problems can result when people "drink" their meals instead of eating nutritious meals.

Anorexia: *The absence or loss of appetite.*

Appetite is the desire to eat certain kinds of food. The *passion* to eat can persist even after hunger or the need for food has been satisfied, as evidenced by the millions of people who are overweight.

Appetite, not to be confused with hunger, is closely associated with the pleasure and enjoyment of eating. Hunger, in contrast, is the physiological drive to satisfy the need for food and energy.

MYTH

Alcohol stimulates appetite.

REALITY

Small amounts of alcohol may stimulate appetite, but in larger quantities, alcohol depresses appetite.

Antabuse (disulfiram): *A prescribed drug used to discourage* *the use of alcohol.* While taking the drug, the individual feels extremely sick if alcohol is consumed.

DID YOU KNOW?

> The use of antabuse during pregnancy is generally not recommended. Women should check with their physician or pharmacist regarding the risks.

Antagonistic effect of drugs: The interaction between drugs where one drug reduces the effect of another drug. (Refer to section on *drug and alcohol interactions.*)

Anxiety: *A state of mind characterized by apprehension, fear, and uneasiness.*

Anxiety can be a major psychological reason for drinking. Since alcohol can immediately reduce tension and stress, the potential for abuse is great.

MYTH

Alcohol reduces anxiety.

REALITY

In small to moderate doses, alcohol has the potential to put the body and mind at ease for a short period of time. However, excessive drinking may actually increase the level of anxiety in many people. More anxiety can lead to more drinking. When more drinking leads to more anxiety, a potentially dangerous cycle begins.

It is important to determine what leads to anxiety. It is important to nip stress and anxiety in the bud, before they become unmanageable. This is not always easy. Learning basic relaxation techniques can help immensely. (Refer to section on *relaxation.*)

Attitude: *Feelings or thoughts that can have an immense effect on behavior and disposition.*

> There is a little difference in people,
> but the little difference makes a big difference.
> The little difference is attitude.
> The big difference is whether
> it is positive or negative.
>
> — *Clement Stone*

Attitudes are rooted in a belief system a person adopts over time. Beliefs are learned and formed from previous experiences. Judgments are made on the *perception* of each experience. It is the evaluation of these experiences that produces a strong feeling or emotion. After an emotion is sparked, an attitude emerges.

Attitudes just don't happen. They unfold and mature.

They are nurtured with personal experience and sustained by belief systems. Attitudes mirror one's feelings and make a direct impact on a person's life. Personality is a reflection of attitudes. Changing one's attitude can change one's life.

> The greatest discovery of my generation is that human beings can alter their lives by altering their attitudes of mind.
>
> — *William James*

Just as attitudes are learned, they can be unlearned. This is great news. It means people can control their destiny by changing negative attitudes. It begins with strengthening the attitude about ourselves. Life is both too short and too long to live with a poor self-image. Alcohol is not a Band-Aid for poor self-esteem. It does not improve one's self-esteem; it only creates a false perception that temporarily modifies one's attitude.

Barbiturates: *Drugs with sedative or hypnotic qualities.* Pentobarbital (Nembutal), secobarbital (Seconal), mobarbital (Amytal), and phenobarbital (Luminal) are common examples of barbiturates. Both psychological and physical dependence or tolerance can develop with the use of barbiturates.

DID YOU KNOW?

The combination of alcohol with any barbiturate is extremely dangerous. It greatly increases the potential for coma and respiratory failure. Too often, alcohol and barbiturates are used together to intensify intoxication.

Beer: *An alcoholic beverage made from malted cereals and hops.* The alcohol content of most beers ranges between three and six percent. Ale, lager, malt liquor and pilsner are examples of different kinds of beers. The caloric value of beer is approximately 13 calories per ounce.

MYTH

The risk of alcohol abuse is greater from drinking hard liquor than from drinking beer.

REALITY

Alcohol is alcohol whether it comes from beer, wine or distilled spirits. Problems can develop from drinking any alcoholic beverage, regardless of its content. Abuse of alcohol, however, is dependent on the dose, frequency and duration of alcohol use, not on the flavor of the drink.

Beliefs: *Beliefs are strong opinions and convictions that influence one's life.* The direction of one's life is determined by a sophisticated belief system. It has the power to both create and destroy. Beliefs control thoughts and actions that determine our future.

> The outer condition of a person's life
> will always be found to reflect their inner beliefs.
>
> —*James Allen*

What beliefs do you have about alcohol? Do you believe that drinking is harmful? Perhaps you believe alcohol is not all that bad. How strong are your beliefs about alcohol? To find out, select the statements in the next chart that accurately reflect your beliefs:

What Are Your Beliefs About Alcohol?

I believe alcohol is:

- ☐ an extremely addicting drug
- ☐ a light to moderately addicting drug
- ☐ not addicting at all

I believe alcohol is:

- ☐ extremely bad for health
- ☐ somewhat bad for health
- ☐ not a health risk
- ☐ good for health

I believe alcohol is:

- ☐ just a part of life and that's the way it is
- ☐ helpful in relaxing and adjusting to stress
- ☐ ruining my life and I need to quit
- ☐ no big deal. I can live with it or without it
- ☐ something I need and can't do without

I believe:

- ☐ I need to question my drinking habits
- ☐ I drink too much
- ☐ I have the power to change

What do you believe?

____

____

____

Binge drinking: *Episodes of excessive drinking.* Drinking habits often do not follow a routine or predictable schedule. Typically, weekends are the favored time for interludes of drinking.

MYTH

Binge drinking is safer than continuous daily drinking.

REALITY

Binge drinking is a form of alcohol abuse. Binge or splurge drinking can be every bit as harmful as chronic drinking. Sometimes it takes only one episode of binge drinking to cause a fatality, injury or permanent disability. Many people choose this method to hide or cope with their drinking habits.

Birth control pills: *A combination of female hormones used as an oral contraceptive to lessen the risk of pregnancy.*

Millions of women take oral contraceptives. Women absorb alcohol more quickly when taking birth control pills. This is also true if they are in the premenstrual phase of their monthly cycle. A more rapid absorption of alcohol can lead to higher blood alcohol levels.

Blackouts: *Episodes of amnesia or memory loss that occur during or after a person has been drinking.* Even though a person's actual consciousness is not lost during a blackout, minutes or several days of their life can be partially or completely "blacked out" or forgotten. Typically, the person who has had a blackout has no recall of events that transpired during a bout with drinking.

Although blackouts are an early warning sign of alcoholism, other signs must also be present. The major symptoms include a heightened tolerance to alcohol and withdrawal sensations if alcohol is not consumed. Keep in mind there are varying degrees of these symptoms.

For years, *heightened* tolerance to alcohol referred to a situation wherein a person required 50 percent more alcohol to achieve the same desired level of intoxication that was previously reached in earlier periods of drinking. Obviously, a certain degree of ambiguity exists with this definition because of the difficulty of determining a precise level of intoxication from consuming 50 percent more alcohol.

The latest criteria used to diagnose alcohol tolerance and dependence can be found in the American Psychiatric Association's *Diagnostic and Statistical Manual (DSM-IV)* in this book's section on *alcohol dependence*.

Blood alcohol concentration (BAC): *The amount of alcohol present in blood.* It is common practice to use blood alcohol levels to determine the degree of a person's alcohol intoxication.

Blood alcohol levels are expressed in milligrams (mg) of alcohol per 100 milliliters (ml) of blood. For convenience, it is easier to refer to blood alcohol concentrations in percentages. A blood alcohol level of 0.05 percent means there are 0.05 grams of alcohol in 100 ml of blood.

DID YOU KNOW?

Alcohol mixes freely with fluids in the body. Therefore, the body fluids in larger individuals dilute alcohol more so than in smaller people. Given two people consuming the same amount of alcohol, the person weighing twice as much will have approximately one-half the blood alcohol level of the smaller person.

Blood-brain barrier: *A protective brain function that screens many harmful substances and prevents them from entering the brain.* Like other psychoactive drugs that alter mood, alcohol is able to cross the blood-brain barrier.

MYTH

It takes 20 minutes for the level of alcohol in the brain to reflect the alcohol level in the blood.

REALITY

Typically, it takes only a few minutes for the brain alcohol level to reflect the level in the blood.

Blood circulation: *The movement of blood through the circulatory or cardiovascular system.* It is responsible for the continuous movement of blood throughout veins and arteries. Blood circulates from deep within the body to the surface of the skin. This marvelous feat is of major importance to the heart and to thousands of miles of intricate blood vessels.

The blood vessels cool the body near the surface of the skin by actually dilating or widening. To conserve heat in cooler weather, the surface blood vessels constrict or shrink in size.

MYTH

In cold weather, alcohol has a warming effect on the body.

REALITY

The consumption of a small amount of alcohol has a subtle effect on a healthy person's circulatory system. There is no significant effect on blood pressure, pulse or blood vessel dilation under these conditions.

Moderate and excessive alcohol intake can lead to vasodilatation (widening) of blood vessels near the surface of the skin. The dilation of these tiny surface blood vessels accounts for the warm or flushed feeling experienced from a few drinks. Despite the pleasant warming sensation, the body is actually losing heat. The same sensation, or heat loss, can be experienced when a person walks into a warm building after being outside in the cold.

Rather than warming the body in the cold, alcohol causes the body to lose heat through the skin. Alcohol should definitely be avoided in cold weather.

Blood glucose: *The sugar found in blood.* The normal level of blood sugar after fasting overnight is between 70 and 115 milligrams per 100 milliliters (one deciliter) of blood. When the blood sugar is too low, a condition called hypoglycemia occurs. A blood sugar level that is too high is called hyperglycemia.

In a hypoglycemic state, a person usually feels lightheaded, hungry, nervous, irritable and weak, and will probably develop a headache.

MYTH

The high sugar content of alcohol helps stabilize blood sugar levels for hypoglycemics.

REALITY

Chemically, alcohol and sugar are worlds apart. Pure alcohol is completely devoid of sugar. Alcohol cannot be converted to sugar in the body. Finally, alcohol inhibits the body's natural ability to make sugar when we have not eaten for awhile. The risk of hypoglycemia is greater for serious drinkers who frequently substitute drinking for eating.

Long gone are the days of whistles and party hats for heavy drinkers. Drinking is a serious business. These people receive excessive calories from alcohol and have little enthusiasm for superfluous energy found in sweet mixers. Although not nutritious, sugary mixers could stave off a bout with hypoglycemia by providing a source of sugar.

Brain atrophy: *Loss of brain cells.* Losing brain cells is nothing like temporarily *losing* your mind such as when you can't find your car keys. Destroying brain cells from alcohol abuse can be a serious problem for heavy drinkers.

Prolonged heavy drinking actually shrinks the size of the brain. The loss of brain cells can occur even before the drinker shows signs of illness. Research suggests that some degree of brain damage from alcohol abuse is reversible if abstinence is maintained.

At higher levels, alcohol can adversely affect oxygen and fuel utilization. Brain cells die when they are deprived of oxygen. Chronic alcohol use causes brain cells to be permanently impaired or lost. Nerve cell transmission and brain cell function are noticeably affected well before permanent brain damage occurs.

MYTH

Only heavy drinking kills brain cells.

REALITY

As the degree of alcohol consumption increases, so too does the level of impairment of brain function and the potential for brain cell loss. There is no clear line separating drinking habits and impairment of brain function. The more a person drinks, the greater the possibility of problems and complications. Every drink slowly chisels away at the size of the brain.

Overall, the risk of brain cell loss and impairment in light to moderate drinkers is quite low. Still, brain function is immediately affected by alcohol, even at low blood alcohol levels.

DID YOU KNOW?

> A person is better able to function when the blood alcohol level is dropping rather than climbing, even when the blood alcohol level is the same.

Breast feeding: *The practice of using the mother's milk to nourish a baby.* Lactation is the production or secretion of milk for the purpose of feeding babies.

MYTH

A mother's milk is protected from alcohol.

REALITY

Is it possible to have had a drink before your first Birthday? Yes. A mother's milk is not immune to alcohol. Any consumption of alcohol while breast feeding will effortlessly find its way into the mother's milk. In essence, the baby will be drinking a *cocktail* while nursing.

Bruising: *The leakage of blood from blood vessels into surrounding tissues following a direct impact injury.*

Drinkers are more prone to bruising or internal bleeding than nondrinkers. Alcohol has a toxic effect on our body's ability to bring bleeding under control after an injury. Normally, blood platelets come racing to the rescue by acting as sticky *tire patches* to put an end to the bleeding. Alcoholics, however, can experience a lower platelet level because alcohol disrupts platelet production in bone marrow. Low platelet levels tend to edge back toward normal levels when the alcoholic takes a sabbatical from drinking for several days.

Caffeine: *A drug found in coffee, tea, cola drinks, and a wide variety of other products.* The stimulant properties of caffeine are well-known by millions who use it to stay alert. It is commonly used to keep eyes open and ears peeled during the waning afternoon hours of a long day.

Just how effective is gulping down a mug or two of coffee after a night of drinking? Let's explore one of the most publicized myths about sobering up with caffeine.

MYTH

Caffeine helps sober up a person who has been drinking.

REALITY

This is wishful thinking. Caffeine has no effect on eliminating alcohol from the body. It can give the drinker a false sense of security since it is a brain or central nervous system stimulant.

The addictive nature of this drug has become all too familiar for those in the caffeine crowd who have tried to abstain from its use. The grip of this household drug on a person's body, however, is nothing like the addictive nature of alcohol. As you can see from the next two tables, caffeine, like alcohol, is found in many different products and has many different effects on the body:

Caffeine Content of Various Beverages and Drugs

Beverages with Caffeine	Caffeine (MG)
Brewed coffee• (1 cup)	80-140
Instant coffee• (1 cup)	60-100
Decaffeinated coffee (1 cup)	1-6
Brewed black tea •(1 cup)	70-110
Instant tea• (1 cup)	30
Cocoa• (1 cup)	10-50
Sanka• (1 cup)	4
Cocoa mix• (1 oz. pkt)	3-16
Soft Drinks (12 oz.)	
Coca-Cola	45
Pepsi-Cola	38
Dr. Pepper	41
Tab	47
Royal Crown Cola	35
Mountain Dew	55
Mr. Pibb	40
Shasta Cola	45
7UP Gold	46
Beverages Without Caffeine	
(7UP, Fresca, root beer, Sprite, Fanta Orange, SunKist Orange, "Caffeine-free")	0
Chocolate Bar* (1 oz.)	25
Common Drugs	(mg/tablet)
Anacin	32
Dristan	30
Excedrin	65
Sinarest	31
Vivarin	100-200
No Doz	100-200
Many cold medicines	30
Darvon	32
Pre-Mens	66
Caferot, many stimulants	100
Midol	32

• Average – caffeine content may vary.

Physiological Effects of Caffeine

Common Effects On the Body

- Does not help sober up an individual
- Central nervous system stimulant
- May arouse drinker
- Temporary decrease in drowsiness and fatigue
- Possible sleep disturbances
- Diuretic (stimulates urine output)
- May make individual anxious
- Stimulates gastric acid secretion
- Stimulates respiration
- Stimulates heart rate
- Vasoconstriction
- Increases blood pressure
- Increases blood glucose and fatty acid levels

Absorption and Metabolism

- Does not increase rate of alcohol oxidation
- Rapidly absorbed by the gastrointestinal tract
- Distributed throughout the body water in about one hour
- Body requires about three hours for one-half to be degraded

Withdrawal Symptoms

- Nausea
- Irritability
- Headaches
- Occasional vomiting

In moderate quantities (approximately 100 mg), caffeine is relatively harmless. Ingestion of larger doses is associated with agitation, restlessness, headaches, intestinal discomfort, dizziness and sleep disorders. The physiological response to caffeine can vary from person to person and from dose to dose.

Calorie: *A unit of energy.* Calories are so small that it takes about 3,500 calories to equal one pound of body fat. Often called a kilo calorie (kcal), the calorie is the easiest way to relate energy with food and drinks.

DID YOU KNOW?

One ounce of alcohol contains

210 Calories

the equivalent of six teaspoons of lard!

Why are excess calories from food and alcohol so fattening? The answer is easy. Look at the table below. Alcohol and fat take first prize for the "High-Energy Fuel Award." They are jammed with calories. From a nutritionist's viewpoint, they furnish calories that cling to our bodies. Wearing large, loose-fitting clothes does little to hide their habitat.

Alcohol commands the liver to make fat at a faster rate. This can be a problem for people who love to eat pizza and drink beer. Incidentally, alcohol does not "cut the grease" in fatty foods.

Energy Value Per Gram of Fuel

• Fat or oils	9 calories
• Alcohol	7 calories
• Carbohydrates	4 calories
• Proteins	4 calories

DID YOU KNOW?

People who consume 2000 calories a day from food are considered heavy drinkers if 10 percent or more of those calories come from alcohol. Exceptionally heavy drinkers obtain more than half of their calories from alcohol.

For most people, five 12-ounce beers typically represent about 25 percent of the caloric intake from alcohol.

To determine the percentage of calories from alcohol in the diet, multiply the grams of alcohol consumed in a day by seven, divide by the total caloric intake for that day, and multiply this number by 100.

Carbohydrates: *One of the main nutrient groups that provides us with energy.* Most of us think of carbohydrates as potatoes, rice, fruits, vegetables, cereals, and soda pop. Alcohol is not a carbohydrate. The effects of carbohydrates and alcohol on the body are worlds apart. As a powerful drug, alcohol has no nutritional value other than providing a rich source of empty calories – something no one needs. On the other hand, carbohydrates should constitute most of our daily food intake.

Carbohydrates found in foods are either sugars or starches. If carbohydrates are sweet, they are *simple* carbohydrates or sugars. If they are not sweet, they are starches, otherwise known as *complex* carbohydrates.

MYTH

Drinkers get many calories from carbohydrates.

REALITY

There are no carbohydrates in alcohol. Most people, whether they drink or not, do not get enough carbohydrates in their diet. At least 60 percent of all the calories or energy we consume each day should come from complex or starchy carbohydrates. Starches, found only in plants, lack the sweet taste of sugar.

DID YOU KNOW?

We should get about five times more energy from starch than from sugar. How can we do this without using a calculator? Simply by cutting down on animal products, eating generous portions of vegetables, breads, beans, rice, cereals or potatoes, and enjoying several helpings of fresh fruit throughout the day. Be creative by dressing up starchy foods with herbs, spices and low fat sauces.

Sweet carbohydrates, or sugars, are good for us when they are found naturally in foods like fruits. The problem with candy, donuts and other "junk" foods is that they are loaded with an abundance of sugar and fat.

People should cut back on sugar and stop eating *empty calorie* foods that displace healthy meals. Consuming high-sugar foods usually means not eating more healthy foods that contain important essential nutrients. Plus, foods high in sugar can be very high in fat. Such diets can aggravate diabetic conditions, promote heart disease and increase the likelihood of developing dental cavities.

There is no doubt that a starch-based carbohydrate diet with some sugar from fruits is the best choice for good physical health.

Carcinogen: *A cancer-causing agent.* The word carcinogen conjures up images of white gowns, hospital beds, and chemotherapy. Alcohol is one of the more infamous carcinogens.

Regular use of alcohol is associated with an increased risk of developing cancer of the mouth, the upper respiratory tract, and the upper gastrointestinal tract. The risk of oral and upper respiratory cancer increases if a person also smokes.

People lucky enough to skirt the odds of incurring cancer will not find comfort in knowing that many other health ailments can surface with continued regular use of alcohol. (Refer to section on *alcohol-related disorders*.)

DID YOU KNOW?

Cancer is a disease characterized by cells that multiply to the point of being out of control.

Cardiac arrhythmia or "Holiday Heart Syndrome": *A fancy term for irregular heartbeat.* Many of us would not mind skipping a few meals now and then, but when it comes to skipping a few heartbeats, the results can be serious.

Whether or not a person has a history of heart disease or alcohol dependence, binge drinking and alcohol abuse can cause abnormalities in cardiac rhythm. This is definitely something to keep in mind at all times, not just during a time of cheer and celebration.

Heavy binge drinking around holidays or weekends has been referred to as the "holiday heart syndrome." The palpitations and irregular heartbeat that characterize this syndrome usually subside with abstinence.

DID YOU KNOW?

The risk of alcohol-related arrhythmias can double in some drinkers who have consumed alcohol equivalent to one bottle of wine.[8]

Cellular tolerance: *A condition whereby the central nervous system or brain becomes less sensitive or responsive to the effect of a drug.*

This condition develops when a person is subjected to the constant assaults of alcohol. A *seasoned* drinker, who needs more alcohol to get the original high, can easily underestimate the degree of physical and mental deterioration from alcohol. Many believe they are better able to handle alcohol with time. In reality, their temporary defense is no match for the impact of excessive alcohol consumption.

In time, the brain suffers the same fate as does the body. It becomes less tolerant and resilient to continued drinking.

DID YOU KNOW?

Older people can become impaired on less alcohol than younger people. Their ability to burn alcohol decreases as they age, so alcohol remains in their bodies longer.

Change: *The modification or transformation of something with the intention to improve.* All of us have the power to change if we believe we can. If we believe we can't, we won't.

> If you think you can,
> or if you think you can't,
> you are right.
>
> — *Henry Ford*

The mere thought that a person can change is one of the simplest thoughts ever entertained. It may be one of the most powerful as well. It requires little effort to hold a thought for a few seconds. Yet the concept of change carries tremendous freedom from self-imposed restraints and limitations.

Change can take as long as a lifetime, or it can take place in a moment. There is awesome power in knowing change begins when a decision is made to do something different. That decision is a huge first step toward realizing personal expectations.

Change is possible when a person knows what to accomplish. There must be specific thoughts and plans.

Undoubtedly, a few tough questions will arise, but they must be answered in as much detail as possible.

Changing thoughts, like changing old habits that no longer serve a person, can be challenging as well as exciting. No one ever said anything worth having didn't have a price tag attached. The trade-off, however, is inconsequential relative to the rewards that can occur when a person makes positive changes in life.

Drinking habits can be changed by writing down a goal, followed by specific action steps. A clear focus eliminates distractions and interferences from old behaviors. (Refer to sections on *goals* and *achievement* for more information.)

MYTH

Once an alcoholic, always an alcoholic.

REALITY

There are two schools of thought on this issue. Some groups, notably Alcoholics Anonymous, support the contention that total abstinence is required to effectively maintain a life of sobriety. Although the debate continues, studies have shown that some reformed alcoholics are able to drink in moderation.

Regardless of the different perspectives, entrenched long-term habits are not easy for the brain to ignore, especially when the roots of a habit are fed by addictive substances. To be safe, a person who decides to stop old destructive habits doesn't need old fires fueled with potential temptations.

Chemical dependence: *Physical and/or psychological reliance on a mood-altering drug.* (See section on *alcohol dependence*.)

DID YOU KNOW?

Nearly one-half of Alcoholics Anonymous members have reported problems or addiction to drugs other than alcohol.[9]

Chronic: *A condition marked by long duration or frequent recurrence.* In contrast, the term *acute* refers to something that develops suddenly and usually lasts a relatively short time.

Individuals who drink on a continuous, long-term basis are referred to as *chronic* drinkers. Chronic alcohol use refers to long-term indulgence, while chronic alcohol *effect* refers to persistent symptoms usually produced by prolonged use of alcohol.

Chronic drinkers who build up a tolerance to alcohol require more and more alcohol to obtain the same effect previously reached. Over time, the brain or central nervous system actually adapts to the presence of alcohol in the early stages of alcoholism. Additionally, habitual drinkers develop an ability to burn alcohol faster. This allows the alcohol to be cleared or removed faster from the body. In the later stage of alcoholism, liver damage can be so severe that alcohol clearance becomes inhibited.

Prolonged drinking can shorten a person's life by many years. Sometimes the end comes instantly. The following table highlights the long-term effects of alcohol use on the body:

Long-Term Effects of Alcohol on The Body

- Impaired immune response
- Nutritional deficiencies leading to malnutrition
- Physical deterioration of organs
  - Fatty liver, alcoholic hepatitis and cirrhosis
  - Alcoholic cardiomyopathy/heart disease
  - Alcoholic myopathy
  - Pancreatitis
- Gastrointestinal ulcers
- Depression and anxiety
- Central nervous system impairment
- Elevated blood pressure
- Increased risk of cancer
  - Mouth, throat, esophagus
- Fetal alcohol syndrome
- Reproductive dysfunction

Cigar Smoke: *The smoke emanating from both ends of a burning cigar.* For some cigar aficionados, cigar lounges and smoke rooms are fast becoming the rival of mocha and coffee cafes across the country. Although most tobacco research has focused on the deleterious effects of cigarette smoke, it is becoming just as certain that cigar smoke is not only addicting and toxic to the human body, but offers the smoker the same risks of oral and throat cancer rates as developed by cigarette smokers who smoke similar amounts of tobacco. A single large cigar can contain as much tobacco as a pack of cigarettes. (Refer to section on *tobacco.*)

MYTH

Cigars contain less nicotine than cigarettes.

REALITY

Some of the larger cigars contain as much as 40 times the nicotine content as a cigarette. Depending on the method of smoking and the size and brand of cigar, cigar smokers may exceed cigarette smokers in their intake of toxins, nicotine, and other cancer causing agents. The nicotine content of cigars can vary greatly, ranging from approximately 10 milligrams to as many as several hundred milligrams of nicotine.

Cigarette smoking: *Inhaling smoke from burning tobacco.* A strong association exists between drinking, smoking, and the risk of developing cancer. Despite warnings, many people play Russian roulette with drinking and smoking. They should ask the question, "Is it really worth the price to play?" (Refer to section on *tobacco.*)

Cirrhosis: *An advanced liver disease in which connective tissue (scar tissue) replaces healthy liver cells.* Permanent damage to liver cells is usually caused by long-term alcohol drinking. For heavy drinkers, cirrhosis can develop in 10 to 15 years. (Refer to section on *liver disease*.)

MYTH

Most alcoholics will eventually develop cirrhosis.

REALITY

Although most heavy drinkers are more likely to suffer from various physiological and psychological problems, cirrhosis is not one of them. Cirrhosis is the final stage of liver disease.

DID YOU KNOW?

A person does not have to be at the "end of the road" before being considered very ill. The liver and body can be in a morbid and unhealthy state and still be cirrhosis-free.

DID YOU KNOW?

Between 15 and 30 percent of alcoholics develop cirrhosis.[10]

African American women between the ages of 15 and 34 are six times, and Native American women are 36 times more likely than Caucasian women to develop cirrhosis of the liver.[11]

Risk of cirrhosis for alcoholic men becomes significant when their average intake of alcohol is about 80 grams of pure alcohol, the equivalent of six 12-ounce beers per day over a 10- to 20-year period. Women are at risk of cirrhosis when they drink about one-quarter of this amount.[12]

Classification of drinking:[13]

Abstainer:

A person who does not consume alcohol. Abstainers don't look to alcohol to alter their mood, impact their life, to celebrate accomplishments, or to deaden the pain of temporary setbacks occasionally dispensed by life.

Light drinker:

The light drinker's average intake of alcohol is no more than 0.22 of an ounce of pure alcohol per day, or five grams of alcohol per day. This is less than one-half of a typical bar drink. Per month, light drinkers consume between one and a dozen drinks.

Moderate drinker:

Many people who think they are light drinkers are actually moderate or even possibly heavy drinkers. Moderate drinkers consume an average of 0.22 to 0.99 ounce of pure alcohol per day. Per week, moderate drinkers consume between four and 13 drinks.

Heavy drinker:

Regardless of sipping or guzzling, the heavy drinker counts on the buzz by consuming an average of 1.0 ounce or more of pure alcohol per day. Per month, heavy drinkers consume the equivalent of 60 drinks or more.

DID YOU KNOW?

One Ounce of Pure Alcohol Equals:

- Two 12-ounce beers
  or
- Two 10-ounce wine coolers
  or
- Two 4-ounce glasses of (12%) wine
  or
- Two 1.25-ounce glasses of distilled spirits

Cocaethylene: *An extremely potent stimulant produced when alcohol and cocaine are used together.* Cocaethylene is significantly more toxic than either cocaine or alcohol alone. It is deadly.

Cocaine: *A powerful mind altering drug that over stimulates the brain and central nervous system.* Processed from the leaves of coca plants, this dangerous and addictive substance is considered by many drug users as the "champagne" of drugs because of its ability to cast an illusion of confidence, power, energy, and well-being over its users.

The artificial sense of euphoria and exhilaration is experienced by the cocaine user until the drug is eventually broken down in the body and the intense high is replaced by a overwhelming low. In many cases, the beginning of cocaine dependence has started well before the user will do almost anything to seek another drug induced high.

MYTH

Cocaine has no side effects.

REALITY

Convulsions, brain seizures, cardiovascular collapse, hypertension, increased heart rate, heart arrhythmia, accelerated respiration, moodiness, sleep disorders, behavioral changes, weight loss, stroke, psychosis, and sudden death are a few notable potential side effects.

MYTH

Long-term use of cocaine
is required to produce addiction.

REALITY

For some people, addiction to cocaine can develop after a few uses, while for others, it may require weeks or months to progress to chemical dependency. All methods employed by users to get the drug into their bodies can produce dependence. Although each form of cocaine is addictive, injecting cocaine or smoking "crack" cocaine can almost instantly create an addiction. People who inject cocaine or share needles to intravenously deliver drugs significantly increase the risk of getting and spreading AIDS and other life-threatening and infectious diseases.

Cold turkey: *Initiating a sudden and complete abstinence from alcohol.*

MYTH

The "cold turkey" method is the best way for an alcoholic to quit drinking.

REALITY

The "cold turkey" method could be disastrous to some alcohol-dependent drinkers without proper medical attention and treatment. The degree of withdrawal symptoms from alcohol deprivation varies. It depends on many factors, including the nature and history of the drinking problem. It is best to seek professional advice and treatment to determine the extent of a person's alcoholism and medical condition.

Confabulation: *A fictional or invented story fabricated by an alcoholic to compensate for actual events that he or she could not remember.*

Congeners: *Chemical substances produced during the process of making alcoholic beverages.* The presence of these organic impurities in alcoholic drinks is thought to contribute to the general malaise or the "hangover" symptoms from overindulgence.

Contraindication: *Any factor in a patient's condition that* *indicates or suggests that it is ill-advised to pursue a specific course of treatment such as surgery or drug therapy.*

There are many reasons why physical and medical records are valuable to doctors. A person's drinking history is just one example. As tough as it may be for some people to be completely honest about their drinking habits, a person's drinking history can provide invaluable information. Medical doctors need this information to avoid any potential contraindications arising from a chosen course of treatment.

Controlled drinking: *The concept of curbed or restricted drinking for an alcoholic.* The idea is based on an alcoholic's ability to drink with restraint and not develop problems with alcohol.

Many groups, including Alcoholics Anonymous, do not support this concept. They advocate that the recovery process for alcoholism must include complete abstention from any source of alcohol for the rest of one's life. (Refer to section of *habits*.)

Cross-tolerance: *A fostered tolerance for other drugs based on a developed tolerance from heavy alcohol drinking*. In effect, the body is demanding a larger dose of certain drugs that will be required to deliver the same punch once rendered. Cross-tolerance is the result of either decreasing the sensitivity of the central nervous system to the drug or increasing the liver's ability to metabolize a drug.

Cross-tolerance between alcohol and other drugs does not occur in every case. Some drugs do not develop an interaction with alcohol. It is especially risky and dangerous to take two drugs at once without knowing the potential for a harmful interaction.

Decisions: *Decisions are steps taken when a commitment is made to resolve or pursue a specific behavior or action.*

One of the biggest decisions a drinker can make is to stop drinking. This does not mean quitting between drinks. Making decisions starts with asking important questions about needs, fears and objectives. Decisions cannot be vague or ambiguous, nor should they be delayed.

> When you know what your values are, making decisions becomes easier.
>
> — *Glen Van Echelon*

Should a person stop drinking? What direction do people want their lives to go? When should they make the change? These questions demand specific answers.

The Art of Making Decisions

Nothing seems to start the ball rolling faster than *making* decisions on what you want to achieve, not about what you have to accept. The direction of a person's life depends on their decisions. When they are resolute about what they want or don't want, or will or will not do, they have then empowered themselves to advance toward their goals and destination.

There is a huge difference between having an interest in something and actually demonstrating an unwavering commitment to it. When someone says, "Gee whiz, I *want* to be rich someday," or "I'd sure like to be in great physical shape," or perhaps, "I need to free myself from drugs," he or she is verbalizing one of two things: It might be a mere interest or curiosity without the necessary commitment to act. On the other hand, they might be saying, "Absolutely nothing will stand in my way. I will get what I want no matter what!"

See the difference? One is a wish. The other is a commitment.

Actually, hundreds of small decisions are made every day with great speed. Some of the quickest decisions are those that people put off. Does the word "procrastination" sound familiar? A decision not to act is still a decision.

When a person makes a decision, it is important to support it with 100 percent effort. It is important not to dwell on other options or look for excuses that abandon decisions. Excuses for not getting started are endless. Writing down short, medium, and long-term goals is helpful to get started.

Certain decisions seem to be a snap, while others are grueling. Why is it that some people can make momentous decisions quickly while others find little decisions a huge undertaking? Generally, decisions are more difficult when a person agonizes over the costs and benefits. How big is the reward? Is there a delay in receiving the reward? How long is the delay? What are the costs? Is there more pain from not doing it, than from doing it?

Taking the Agony Out of Making Decisions

- Focus on what is important

Decisions are made with less effort when a person knows what is important. It can be done by making a list of values and ranking them in order of importance. This becomes the "weighing system." Committing to decisions that support high-ranking values is a key element of success.

- Take a load off the mind.

Many people roll questions around in their minds for literally years and never find answers. At times, this *indecision* is enough to drive a person crazy. For relief, a person needs to begin by getting unsettled business out of their head. Writing down ideas and thoughts renders those thoughts highly visible, ready to organize, and act upon.

- Weigh the difference.

Decisions are made more easily when a person knows how much they have to pay for the *goods* they want. Anything worth having has some cost. The question becomes, "What am I willing to pay?" Any person who would like to make an important decision about drinking could use the next table to help sort out the costs and benefits:

Costs and Benefits of Drinking

Identify all the benefits and rewards from drinking.

____

____

____

____

____

____

____

Identify all costs, losses, and suffering from drinking.

____

____

____

____

____

____

____

____

____

____

Delirium tremens (DTs): *A severe withdrawal reaction from alcohol characterized by fever, nausea, severe agitation, and uncontrolled violent muscle contractions.* Additional symptoms include trembling, convulsions, hallucinations, terror, and varying degrees of mental confusion. These symptoms usually last several days before subsiding. As a general rule, the withdrawal process usually lasts several days to a week.

Proper medical attention for more serious conditions will minimize the risk of further complications during the DTs. (For more information, refer to section on *withdrawal*.)

Denial: *A clever method used by alcoholics to renounce or deny that they have a drinking problem.* It may seem ridiculous that alcoholics could deny that a problem is harming them, and everything in its path, but it happens time and again. Careers, families and homes are just a few examples of casualties that mount in the wake of denial.

Ordinarily, we could not watch a home or building burn to the ground and then reject that it ever happened. But alcoholics slowly watch themselves destroy their mind, body, spirit, and soul while in a state of complete denial. Sadly, many people do this!

With denial, foolishness and fantasy replace reasoning and reality. The result is crippling and destructive not only to those in denial, but also to the loved ones who are closest to them.

Detoxification: *Considered the initial phase of a drug abuse treatment program where sufficient time is allowed to eliminate* *all traces of a drug from the body.*

If the body has adjusted to a long-term heavy drinking schedule, a sudden suspension of drinking can cause severe withdrawal symptoms and potential death. In less advanced stages of alcoholism, withdrawal may be less dangerous and may not require medical assistance.

It is important to know the risk before making a sudden change in drinking habits. Call for information or assistance. (Refer to *resource information guide* for assistance.)

Diabetes: *A disease or disorder in which insufficient amounts of insulin are produced after a meal or the insulin that is produced is ineffective.* In other words, insulin is not doing the job it was instructed to do. The movement of sugars from the blood into body cells is the primary job of insulin.

Clinically, there are two types of diabetes. Type I diabetes, also called insulin-dependent, growth-onset, or juvenile-onset, is much less common than Type II diabetes.

Type II diabetes, also called noninsulin-dependent, maturity-onset, or adult-onset, represents the most prevalent form of diabetes. About 80 percent of diabetics fall into this category. Type II diabetes is characterized by insulin resistance.

Some physiological symptoms of an untreated diabetic include hyperglycemia, glycosuria (glucose in the urine), polyuria (frequent urination), polydipsia (increased fluid intake), weight loss, and ketosis.

Drinking and diabetes

In many cases, small doses of alcohol consumed with food do not seem to disrupt blood sugar levels in diabetics. This holds true only if the diabetic's condition is under control at the time. Depending on the type and severity of the diabetic's condition, proper diet, drug treatment and/or insulin may be needed to avoid high blood sugar or hyperglycemic states. Ingesting alcohol with *oral insulin,* containing sulfonyl derivatives, may produce a drug alcohol interaction causing nausea and dizziness.

Moderate to excessive amounts of alcohol can cause problems in diabetics, especially if the drinks contain sugar or if the diabetic is drinking on an empty stomach. Alcohol on an empty stomach often leads to hypoglycemia or low blood sugar. This becomes a potential problem for the diabetic. Alcohol interferes with the body's natural ability to make glucose (sugar) in the unfed state and can cause blood sugar levels to fall.

Combining alcohol with food can have the reverse effect, producing a hyperglycemic condition. Diabetics and people with problems stabilizing blood sugar levels need to think twice before drinking that may send them on a roller coaster blood sugar ride.

Digestion: *The process of preparing and converting food into a form suitable for absorption by the body.* Alcohol does not need to be digested before it is absorbed into the blood system.

MYTH

Alcohol helps digest food.

REALITY

For some people, enjoying a small glass of wine before dinner may play a minor role in the overall picture of digestion. However, most people will do just fine without any assistance from alcohol in promoting the flow of digestive juices within the stomach. A healthy body is equipped to dismantle the thousands of different foods we eat. The best digestive aid is simply to eat well.

In larger quantities, alcohol may actually become an irritant to the lining of the stomach; consequently, it would be the last choice to help in the digestive process. Intoxicating quantities of alcohol interfere with digestion.

> Many a man keeps on drinking
> 'til he hasn't a coat to either
> his back or his stomach.
>
> — George D. Prentice

Disease: *Any abnormal or unhealthy condition or process in which normal biochemical or physiological function is disrupted.*

Although certain infections or diseases seem to be unavoidable at times, certain steps can be taken to bolster a natural defense against illnesses. (Refer to section on *immune system* for more information.)

Distress: *Distress is another word for "bad stress."* It is a killer in disguise. Aside from being unpleasant, it is a major factor in triggering the abuse of alcohol. Millions of people seek its use to ease or temporarily escape pain. By reducing the degree of distress, the urge to drink usually subsides. (For more detail, refer to section on *stress*.)

If you are distressed by anything external,
the pain is not due to the thing itself,
but to your own estimate of it;
and this you have the power
to revoke at any moment.

— *Marcus Aurelius*

DID YOU KNOW?

Anxiety, depression, and stress are just a few factors that motivate certain people to abuse alcohol.

Diuretic: *A chemical substance that causes increased urine flow or excretion from the body.* Alcohol is a diuretic. When we lose too many fluids, dehydration can become a serious problem. A hefty thirst is the first sign that the body has lost fluids that need to be replaced immediately. Otherwise, muscles will surrender much of their strength and endurance. The seriousness of the situation will escalate with further fluid loss.

Alcoholic beverages may seem like a source for needed fluids, but alcohol is a villain in disguise. Acting as a diuretic, alcohol actually instructs the kidneys to "pull the plug," sending a person on another trip to the rest room.

Physically active people who sip alcoholic drinks in warm and hot climates should be aware of the significant risk of fluid loss and overheating. Staying hydrated includes drinking sufficient water or your favorite fruit juice.

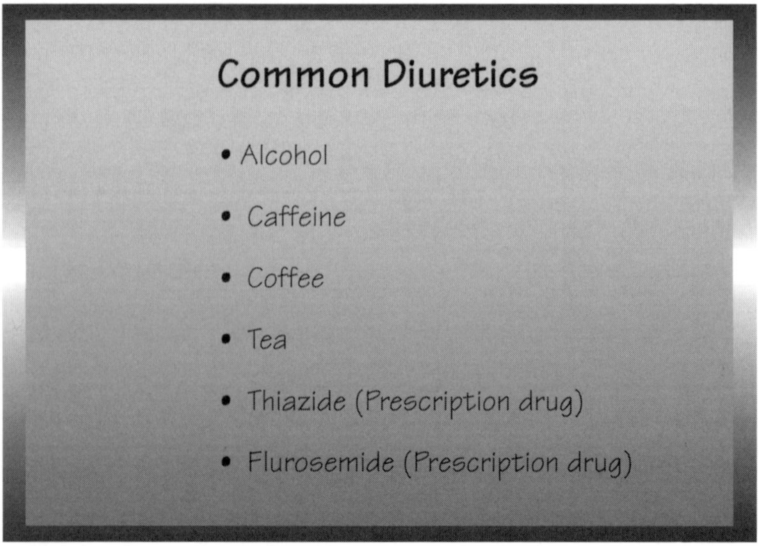

Driving under the influence (DUI): *Driving a motor vehicle while under the influence of an intoxicating drug.* Let's make an unequivocal point about drinking and driving: few things can be as foolish as becoming intoxicated and getting behind the wheel.

The number of senseless highway accidents and deaths related to alcohol use is staggering, yet these statistics do little to dissuade some people from "taking chances."

By checking with the local Highway Patrol, people can determine the legal limit for blood alcohol levels while driving. In many cases, 0.08 percent blood alcohol or less constitutes driving under the influence; however, a blood alcohol concentration below the legal intoxication level does not ensure risk-free driving.

There is no safe way to drive after drinking. Even one drink can make you an unsafe driver. Drinking affects your BLOOD ALCOHOL CONCENTRATION (BAC). It is illegal to drive with a BAC of .08 percent (.04 percent if you have a commercial driver license or .01 percent or more if under age 21). Even a BAC below .08 percent does not mean it is safe or legal to drive. The charts on the next page show the BAC zones for various numbers of drinks and time periods.

HOW TO USE THESE CHARTS: Find the chart that includes your weight. Look at the total number of drinks you have had and compare that to the time shown. You can quickly tell if you are at risk of being arrested. If your BAC level is in the gray zone, your chances of having a collision are five times higher than if you had no drinks, and 25 times higher if your BAC level falls into the black zone.

REMEMBER: "Onc drink" is a 12-ounce beer, or a four-ounce glass of wine, or a one-ounce shot of 80-proof liquor (even if it's mixed with nonalcoholic drinks). If you have larger or stronger drinks, or drink on an empty stomach, you can be UNSAFE with FEWER drinks. Also, you can be unsafe with fewer drinks if you are tired, sick, upset, or have taken medicines or drugs.

TECHNICAL NOTE: These charts are intended to be guides and are not legal evidence of the actual blood alcohol concentration. Although it is possible for anyone to exceed the designated limits, the charts have been constructed so that fewer than five persons in 100 will exceed these limits when drinking the stated amounts on an empty stomach. Actual values can vary by body type, sex, health status, and other factors.

Adapted and reprinted with permission from the California State Department of Motor Vehicles.

STATE OF CALIFORNIA
0.08 % DUI CHARTS
DRINKING ALCOHOL AND DRIVING AT ANY AGE IS ILLEGAL

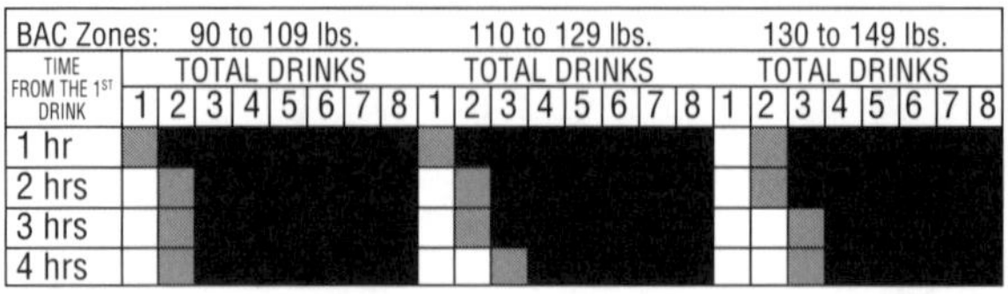

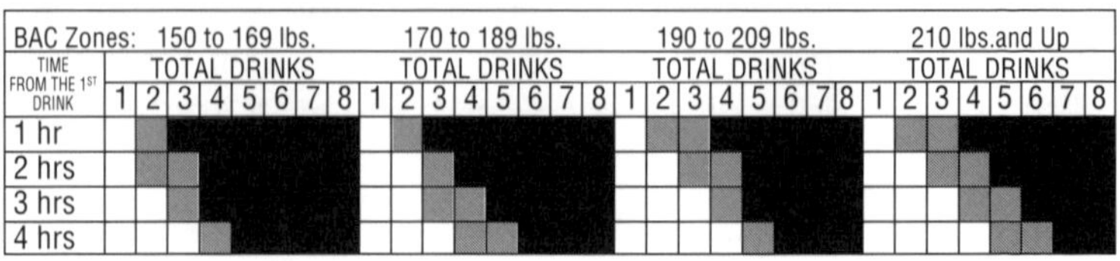

SHADING IN THE CHARTS ABOVE MEAN:

- ☐ (.01%-.04%) May be DUI–*DEFINITELY DUI IF UNDER 21 YRS. OLD*
- ▒ (.05%-.07%) Likely DUI–*DEFINITELY DUI IF UNDER 21 YRS. OLD*
- ■ (.08% Up) Definitely DUI

DID YOU KNOW?

The risk of dying from an automobile wreck is 11 times greater for drivers with a blood alcohol concentration (BAC) between 0.05 and 0.09 percent. The risk is nearly 50 times greater when the blood alcohol level is between 0.10 and 0.15 percent. With a blood alcohol level above 0.15 percent the risk increases almost 400 times.[14]

Nearly 50 percent of automobile accidents are associated with alcohol use.[15]

Nearly 50 percent of all highway fatalities are alcohol-related.[16]

Drug: *A drug is any chemical substance that alters the function of a body process.*

Drugs used for medicinal value are prescribed or obtained "over-the-counter." Drugs that are not intended for specific medical use are usually considered social or recreational drugs. Alcohol is a prime example of a "social" drug. Millions of people use alcohol to relax, celebrate, escape, or alter the perception of their environment.

Drugs are usually given three different names: a descriptive chemical name, a generic name, and a brand name. Drugs are classified according to chemical makeup or identity; specific biological effects on the body; or the disease/disorder they are intended to treat.

Many drugs have important functions in medicine. They are used to treat, prevent, or reduce the severity of symptoms caused by a disorder. Drugs stimulate or inhibit chemical processes. As a drug, alcohol affects many of these processes.

The next table itemizes a small list of commonly abused drugs:

Depressants:

- Alcohol (ethanol, "ethyl alcohol," "grain alcohol")
- Barbiturates (amytal, nembutal, phenobarbital, seconal)
- Benzodiazepines (valium, librium, halcion, xanax)
- Chloral hydrate (noctec)

Stimulants:

- Amphetamine (dexedrine, methamphetamine, "speed," "crank")
- Cocaine ("coke," "crack")
- Methylphenidate (ritalin)

Narcotics:

- Codeine, demerol, heroin, methadone, morphine, opium

Drug addiction: *Uncontrollable desire or chronic craving for a particular substance.* Addiction can be physical, psychological, or both. Drug dependence, another term for drug addiction, includes the use of a drug for a desired effect or to eliminate ill effects resulting from its abstinence. A problem clearly develops when there is an uncontrollable desire or chronic craving for a particular substance.

Let's look at the difference between psychological and physiological dependence. Someone develops a *psychological* dependence when that person continues to use a particular drug to thwart cravings, prevent uneasiness and to avoid emotional distress. *Physical* dependence has developed when, upon elimination of the drug, the body experiences severe physical and mental withdrawal symptoms.

A dependence on alcohol and other addicting drugs usually develops as a result of excessive and/or regular use of a drug over some period of time. An occasional bout with alcohol takes on more significance when drinking becomes routine. When people nurture drinking habits, they add insult to injury. The road to dependence is built on one drink at a time. (Refer to section on *alcohol dependence.*)

Drug and alcohol interactions: *The effect or result of combining one or more drugs with alcohol.* Since the liver plays an extremely important role in metabolizing drugs other than alcohol, potentially dangerous alcohol-drug interactions can occur in both light and heavy drinkers. The possibility for problems abounds with thousands of prescription and nonprescription drugs/medications on the market. Many commonly prescribed drugs are known to interact with alcohol.

The physical consequences of an alcohol-drug interaction depend on:

- amount of alcohol present in the body
- type and quantity of medication or drugs used
- the person's age, sex, and health
- the person's drinking record

DID YOU KNOW?

> Many older drinkers are at greater risk of alcohol-drug interactions if they are taking medications. As we get older, the likelihood of requiring medications to treat age-related illnesses and diseases increases.

An interaction between alcohol and a drug is described as any change in the properties or effects of either drug in the presence of the other. Drug interactions may be:

- **Additive – the net effect of the drugs taken together is the sum of the effects of the individual drugs; in other words, one plus one equals two.**

- **Antagonistic – the effect of either or both drugs are diminished in the presence of each other.**

- **Supra additive – the effect of the drug combination is greater than the sum effects of the two drugs; in other words, one plus one is greater than two.**

The MEOS System for Drug Metabolism

One way the body breaks down alcohol is through the action of specialized proteins called enzymes. These enzymes begin dismantling the alcohol soon after it is consumed. Typically, they can handle alcohol under light to moderate drinking conditions.

Heavy or "marathon" drinking requires the deployment of additional enzyme forces to deal with the inventory of surplus alcohol. The long, unattractive name, microsomal ethanol-oxidizing system, inherits the nickname MEOS system. This enzyme system deserves huge praise for its role in assisting drinkers who are recovering from overindulgence. The MEOS system actually matures and becomes more effective as a person's drinking habits become more entrenched with time. The light drinker has little need for this system.

Potential problems with drug interactions occur due to differences in drinking habits. The MEOS system can become overwhelmed if it has to work with more than one drug at a time, especially if the MEOS system is not induced or "powered up." Compare this with trying to catch two balls at the same time while one hand is tied behind your back. One ball, or drug, is "missed." The potential for drug toxicity increases if it is not removed or broken down at the intended rate.

On the other hand, excessive drinking over a period of time can speed up the MEOS system. The body may not receive an intended drug dose because it is being metabolized too quickly.

Using two or more drugs at once can cause the *additive* effects to occur. When two drugs are taken together, the combined effects can be much different than expected. In other words, one plus one can equal three or four. Multiple use of drugs is not recommended unless prescribed by a physician for a specific use.

Drug interaction problems can arise from carelessness. It is important to seek advice and information from a doctor or pharmacist about possible drug interactions with alcohol.

DID YOU KNOW?

> Drug interactions differ significantly between light and heavy drinkers. Of particular concern is the use of alcohol and psychotropic drugs (drugs that alter behavior or mood). Sometimes these drugs are called *psychoactive* in keeping with their impact on the brain or central nervous system. Alcohol should not be used in combination with any of these drugs.
>
> Antidepressant, antianxiety, and antipsychotic represent the three major categories of psychotropic drugs.

The following charts represent a partial list of some of the commonly prescribed drugs that should not be mixed with alcohol:

Antidepressant Drugs
(used to treat depression)

Drugs that should not be mixed with alcohol

Brand name	Generic name
Elavil	Amitriptyline
Pamelor	Nortriptyline
Paxil	Paroxetine
Prozac	Fluoxetine
Tofranil	Imipramine
Zoloft	Sertraline
MAOI	
Nardil	Phenelzine
Parnate	Tranylcypromine

Note: The combination of alcohol, MAOIs, and tyramine (found in aged cheese and in some alcoholic beverages, such as Chianti wine), can lead to high blood pressure and convulsions.

Hypnotic/Tranquilizing Drugs

(used to induce sleep)

Drugs that should not be mixed with alcohol

Brand name	Generic name
Ativan	Lorazepam
Equanil	Meprobamate
Librium	Chlordiazepoxide
Serax	Oxazepam
Tranxene	Clorazepate
Valium	Diazepam

Note: These drugs are often called minor tranquilizers. The potential for abuse in combination with or without alcohol can be high.

Antianxiety Drugs

(used to produce sedation and tranquilization)

Drugs that should not be mixed with alcohol

Brand name	**Generic name**
Ambien	Zolpidem
Dalmane	Flurazepam
Halcion	Triazolam
Restoril	Temazepam

Note: These drugs are used to induce sleep. They can interact with alcohol to potentiate or increase the effect of the drug.

Antipsychotic Drugs

(used to treat psychosis, and occasionally as a sedative)

Drugs that should not be mixed with alcohol

Brand name	Generic name
Haldol	Haloperidol
Loxitane	Loxapine
Mellaril	Thioridazine
Navane	Thiothixene
Prolixin	Fluphenazine
Stelazine	Trifluoperazine
Thorazine	Clorpromazine
Trilafon	Perphenazine

Note: These drugs are often called major tranquilizers or neuroleptics. They can interact with alcohol to potentiate or increase the effect of the drug.

DSM-IV: *The American Psychiatric Association's fourth edition of the Diagnostic and Statistical Manual, used as a standard for naming and distinguishing psychiatric disorders.*

Dysphoria: *A malaise associated with withdrawal or hangovers.*

Enabling: *A pattern of behavior by family or close friends that accommodates or "protects" the drinker.* The enabler inadvertently supports drinking by making excuses or overlooking the seriousness of the problem.

Making excuses, downplaying the seriousness of a drinking problem, or not admitting a problem is present only kindles a drinker's flare for denial. The drinker should be made aware that a problem clearly exists and that continued drinking will not be accepted or tolerated. This is most effective if done without berating or nagging the drinker.

The drinker needs love, support and encouragement in exploring the benefits of professional guidance.

Energy: *The fuel we derive from food and beverages.* Foods or beverages high in calories and low in nutrients are often called "junk" or "empty" calorie foods. Healthy bodies do not run well on poor quality fuels, and alcohol is just that, a poor quality fuel.

Although alcohol contains many calories, it has zero nutritional value. Moreover, alcohol is known to increase the need for certain nutrients. It has a damaging effect on the absorption of key nutrients and can cause the premature and unwanted excretion of some nutrients.

MYTH

Alcohol is a rich source of energy for muscles to burn.

REALITY

Although alcohol is a rich source of energy, muscles are not able to burn alcohol. Muscles also despise proteins as a source of energy. Their usual menu is composed of sugars and fats. An alternate fuel, known as *ketone bodies*, supplies muscles with energy during times of food shortages.

Although the liver is the major site for alcohol oxidation, a significant amount of alcohol can be burned in the stomach. Gastric oxidation of alcohol is significantly slower for women. Regardless of where it is burned in the body, alcohol is always high in energy.

DID YOU KNOW?

Some alcoholics consume as much as one-half of their energy needs from alcohol.[17]

Environment: *The physical, mental, social, and spiritual world in which a person lives.*

As a general rule, if people are not happy with their environment, they need to change it.

Dismal thoughts are breeding grounds for depression and drinking. To change any aspect of our environment, we can begin by lifting our attitude by concentrating on our positive qualities. We all have a negative and positive side to our character; the trick is to find the bright side and hold on to it.

Culture plays a significant role as well. Availability of alcohol can promote the consumption of alcoholic beverages. Its social acceptance at home, in restaurants, airports, ball games, and after-work gatherings presents enticing surroundings. Drinking can become a way of spending or passing time in these settings. Having assorted juices and nonalcoholic beverages available allows people to have another option.

Stressful environments cannot be changed by drinking. They can, however, be increased because the root problems are not addressed. If people are drinking to survive or to cope with a stressful environment, they might benefit by focusing on practical solutions that offer realistic outcomes.

Exercise and drinking: *Exercise involves activities that require the use of various muscle groups.* Alcohol is not a good fuel for exercise. Despite alcohol's rapid absorption into the body and its rich source of energy, it cannot be burned for energy by muscles. (Refer to the section on *energy*.)

Muscles burn sugars and fats. Sugars are primarily used as a source of energy during *anaerobic* workouts or activities that make it difficult to catch a breath of air. During *aerobic* workouts, where people are not laboring as hard to breathe, they burn more fat.

Regardless of the ratio of sugar to fat being burned, muscles need a certain supply of sugar. The body produces some of this sugar from the degradation of stored carbohydrates in the liver and muscle. It can maintain the supply for up to about 90 minutes during extensive workouts. As these sugar or "glycogen" stores are depleted, the liver makes every attempt to replenish them.

The saga of alcohol and exercise unfolds in stages. Alcohol slices the fuel lines to the muscles in two spots. Alcohol cannot be metabolized or converted to sugar, as it interferes with the liver's ability to make sugar for energy use. As the blood sugar level drops, the risk of hypoglycemia goes up and physical endurance goes down.

In most cases, the recommended diet for the athlete or nonathlete is the same: a variety of plant or starchy foods low in fat. Many people become victims of fads, misconceptions and poor advice about diet and exercise. Advertisements proclaiming miraculous health and physical benefits from taking "sports supplements" may be misleading and/or inappropriate for the generally active person. Most active people do not require additional nutrients beyond those obtained in a balanced diet.

Although athletes have higher nutritional needs, they are easily met by eating nutritious foods that support energy requirements for physical activity.

The following information is a basic nutritional guide:

Nutritional Guide For Physical Activity

- Avoid the use of alcoholic beverages before, during, and after exercise.

- Increase the quantity of nutritious foods that supply extra energy needed for physical activities. Refer to *nutrition* section for details.

- Replace fluids ("rehydration") during and after a strenuous event.

Athletes can easily lose two to four quarts of water per hour during heavy exercise. An adequately hydrated body, before a sports event, is equally important. The body absorbs about one liter, or quart, of water per hour. It is essential that the athlete keep hydrated with water during and after the event.

Excessive water and electrolyte loss will impair heat tolerance and physical performance. It can lead to heat cramps, exhaustion, fatigue, and possibly heat stroke. The time to be concerned about water replacement is during and after the exercise.

Fat and drinking: *Excess weight resulting from insufficient exercise and the consumption of too much food and/or alcoholic beverages.* This excess weight is commonly referred to as "rolls," "tires," "flab," or "buns."

Also known as adipose tissue, body fat never goes out of style. It is worn year-round, rain or shine. The fat you cannot see is the ugliest of all. It lines the arteries and can build up until the flow of nutrients and oxygen to the heart becomes blocked. Washing rich, fatty meals down the gullet with booze will neither "cut" the fat nor contribute to a healthy life-style.

DID YOU KNOW?

A person gains approximately one pound of body fat for every 3,500 excess calories consumed from foods or beverages.

The following tips will help trim the fat out of a diet:

Tips for Reducing Fat In the Diet

- Read food labels — Purchase nonfat or low-fat foods.
- Steam, boil or bake foods. Avoid frying foods.
- Restrict intake of baked goods such as biscuits, croissants, doughnuts, rolls, and chips.
- Use fat-free salad dressings.
- Eliminate the "meat-based diet." Make rice, vegetables, potatoes, beans, etc. the focus of meals.
- Eat fruit for dessert without ice-cream or whipped cream toppings.
- Cut or spoon off visible fat from cooked or uncooked foods.
- If purchasing meat, select the leanest cuts possible.
- Use nonstick frying pans with a small amount of vegetable spray.
- Season foods with herbs and spices rather than with butter, margarine or salt.
- Prepare meatless sauces.
- Select foods packed in water rather than oils.
- Use two egg whites in place of one whole egg in recipes that call for eggs.
- Use skim or low-fat milk rather than whole milk in recipes that call for milk.

Fatty liver: *An early stage of liver disease characterized by an accumulation of fat in the liver.* Fatty liver is characterized by blotchy yellow streaks of fat that slowly destroy the liver. Hopefully, the sight of this "poisoned" organ will make anyone think twice about abusing alcohol.

Clearing the liver of fat can be accomplished in the early stages of a drinking habit if the person adheres to a healthy diet and abstains from alcohol.

DID YOU KNOW?

Given similar drinking habits, women are more likely to have liver disease than men.[18,19]

Fear: *A frightening emotion that can cripple or paralyze a person from taking action.* Fear is a distressing emotional state. It is evoked by anticipation of danger, pain, loss or change, whether real or imagined. Most fear is based on two things: the uncertainty associated with change and a lack of confidence in dealing with the unfamiliar.

Roots that feed fear are embedded in insecurity. Fear has no boundaries. People can fear just about anything: aging, speaking, dancing, thinking, or just *ordinary* living. Millions of people abuse alcohol to deaden the suffering resulting from uncertainty. Drinking only temporarily shelters a person from fear.

In order for people to free themselves of fear, they must

challenge fear head-on, without alcohol. They must be willing to step outside their "comfort spheres," that haven or sanctuary where things seldom change or improve. This sphere serves as an asylum where wishing and longing replace action and results.

In the most difficult times, when a person is feeling the most insecure and vulnerable, the biggest and most rewarding changes can take place. By confronting fear, anyone can refuse to be blinded by its facade.

> *Some of your hurts you have cured,*
> *and the sharpest you still have survived,*
> *but what torments of grief you endured,*
> *from evils that never arrived.*
>
> *—Ralph Waldo Emerson*

Fermentation: *A biological process by which enzymes convert carbohydrates into alcohol in yeast cells.* Imagine what human life would be like if we had such enzymes in our bodies! A sobering thought.

Alcohol is produced from a biological process called fermentation. Via the fermentation process, yeast cells convert the carbohydrates of plants such as fruits, grains, or potatoes, into alcohol. However, these tiny yeast cells do have limits. They will only produce alcohol and survive until the alcohol content reaches 14 percent.

The production of "spirits" or more potent alcoholic beverages from fermented products is easily accomplished by distillation. This process separates the alcohol content of a fermented product by removing the water. Approximately 95 percent alcohol level can be obtained if enough water is removed through the distillation process. Since alcohol will dilute itself by mixing with moisture in the air, it is not possible to attain 100 percent alcohol.

Fetal alcohol syndrome (FAS): *A combination of mental and physical abnormalities present in infants born to mothers who consumed alcohol during pregnancy.*

MYTH

One to two alcoholic drinks
a day during pregnancy is safe.

REALITY

A mother's body cannot protect the embryo/fetus from even small amounts of alcohol. Any consumed alcohol is freely passed by the mother's blood into her baby's system.

The level of alcohol in an unborn baby's blood is at least as high as that of the mother's blood. Before, during, and after pregnancy, it is critical to be drug and alcohol-free unless a specific medication is prescribed by a licensed medical doctor.

Potential FAS Symptoms

- Brain changes
  - small brain
  - mental retardation
  - poor coordination
- Organ defects
  - heart
  - urinary system
  - genitals
  - ears
  - cleft palate
- Deformed facial features
  - wide-set eyes
  - flattened nose
- Joint deformities
- Growth retardation
- Behavioral changes
  - hyperactivity
  - sleep disorders

What is a safe drinking level for a pregnant woman?

Thousands of scientific reports prove that alcohol can cause lifelong defects in children born to mothers who consumed alcohol during pregnancy.

Alcohol increases the risk of miscarriage, decreased birth weight, or a permanently harmed child. A major challenge facing scientists today is to uncover and correlate subtle injuries caused by variable drinking habits of pregnant women.

FAE, otherwise known as Fetal Alcohol Effects, represents defects in children who were not severely impaired with overt physical deformities. Physical agility, behavioral abnormalities, and slow learning are examples of FAE. They are all too frequently the telltale signs of a mother who drank excessively during pregnancy.

There is no conclusive evidence about how much alcohol is required to cause the physical and mental problems associated with Fetal Alcohol Syndrome. Subsequently, the U.S. Surgeon General, American Medical Association and other health authorities, strongly recommend that no alcohol be consumed during pregnancy.

DID YOU KNOW?

The risk of Fetal Alcohol Syndrome (FAS) is about seven times higher in African American women than in Caucasian women.[20]

DID YOU KNOW?

- Binge drinking is especially dangerous during the first three months of pregnancy.
- Poor diet, cigarette smoking, stress, and the use of other drugs compounds FAS-related problems.
- Avoid alcohol consumption when trying to conceive. Many women are unaware of their pregnancy during the first two to three months.
- It takes about 15 minutes for the fetal blood alcohol level to rise to mother's blood alcohol level. The effects of blood alcohol on the mother and fetus are, however, strikingly different. The detoxification system is much less developed in the unborn child. An hour of binge drinking during critical periods of pregnancy can be devastating.

DID YOU KNOW?

Economic losses related to Fetal Alcohol Syndrome cost our society billions of dollars each year.[21]

Fortified wines: *Wines to which alcohol has been added.* Fortified wines include: Sherry, Madeira, Marsala, Vermouth, and Port wines. Fortified wines average about 20 percent alcohol.

Genetic inheritance: *The "bundle of traits" or genetic characteristics passed from parents to their children.*

DID YOU KNOW?

> Research studies have revealed a genetic link regarding the susceptibility to alcoholism.[22]

It is common knowledge that alcoholism runs in certain families. Inheriting alcoholic traits is one of several causes for alcoholism. Human and animal research supports this thinking.

The real question is not whether genetics plays a role in alcoholism, but rather, to what extent? There is no doubt that certain physical traits are passed on from one generation to another. This inherited genetic endowment determines what biological instructions will be used in a person's physical development.

Genetic instructions, coupled with environmental factors such as nutrition, exercise, stress, drug education, and life-style choices, work together to influence a predisposition to drink. Research studies have revealed a genetic link regarding the susceptibility to alcoholism.[22]

The degree to which cultural, physical, emotional, and environmental factors contribute to drinking will probably be debated for years. The only certainty is that the motivation for drinking will continue to vary between individuals and situations.

Glycemic index: *A system that ranks foods according to how they change blood glucose levels.* The *glycemic effect,* sometimes referred to as *glycemic response*, refers to the effect a particular food or drink, such as alcohol, has on the blood sugar level and insulin response. Insulin *response* refers to the amount of insulin released into the blood following a meal.

Generally, complex carbohydrates (starches) elicit a weaker glycemic response than simple carbohydrates (sugars). The glycemic effect of food also depends on whether it is a liquid, solid, paste, or cooked. The type and amount of fiber, fat, protein, and carbohydrates present are other contributing factors.

Although alcohol has virtually no effect on insulin release, diabetics and hypoglycemics may want to think twice about drinking alcohol, because alcohol, in other ways, disrupts carbohydrate metabolism.

Goals: *Organized plans, or "targets," that help people focus their attention.* Goals encompass objectives, agendas, and/or mission statements. Achieving a goal, however, depends on commitment, dedication, and intense concentration. Hazy, vague goals produce fuzzy results. People who have difficulty reaching goals may not have taken the time to visualize them.

A goal can become reality with just a few small steps. Goals remain empty aspirations and unfulfilled dreams without direction and action.

Eight key rules for setting goals and reshaping behavior are presented below. Together, they have the power to change destructive drinking or other harmful habits. Read them and hang them on the refrigerator.

> Far away in the sunshine are my highest
> aspirations. I may not reach them,
> but I can look up and see their beauty,
> believe in them, and try to follow where they lead.
>
> — *Louisa May Alcott*

Key Goal Setting Rules

Rule 1 — Identify a desire or need.

Do goals involve personal growth, work, leisure, relationships, finances, health or fitness? Specific interests need to be identified.

> Things which matter most must never
> be at the mercy of things which matter least.
>
> — *Goethe*

Rule 2 — Identify what gets in the way of changing.

Sometimes we blame other people for preventing us from accomplishing a certain goal. The truth is, we are usually our own worst interference. We don't need anyone to stop us; we can do it ourselves. How many silent conversations have you had with yourself that limit and block change? Some people have them daily. This private "chatterbox" can shackle a person to the same old way of thinking. Every day, some people play negative tapes about doubt, insecurity, pity, and worry.

Changing this pattern requires silencing the negative chatter. Recognize what tape is playing, then eject it and insert a new, more positive voice.

Rule 3 — Make sure change needs to happen.

Time is truly a precious commodity. Most people do not think about the value of time until reminded by a birthday, a deadline, or death itself. Before spending valuable time designing a goal, be certain it is something truly needed. Many times we labor over things that are unimportant or we do what other people want.

Be clear about what is valued. If good health is the goal, outline steps that will accomplish this. If drinking habits prevent pleasure, then the goal becomes "stop drinking." A first step might be to get the liquor out of the house. Simply declining a routine glass of wine at dinner is another important step.

Rule 4 — Goals must be specific.

It feels great to have lofty goals. Although they help us aim in the right direction, such goals can be too abstract to manage.

People who simply want to be "healthy, wealthy, and wise,"

need to divide these goals into specific objectives.

Tangible steps toward improving health could mean reaching a target blood pressure, cholesterol level, or resting heart rate. It could also mean specifying a desired weight or gaining freedom from medications or drugs used to treat a specific condition. Saying NO MORE to smoking, drinking, and eating rich, fatty foods are also examples of setting specific goals.

Let's say we would like to be more physically fit. Whether we want to walk upstairs without getting winded or run a marathon race, we must be specific and picture our goal in detail.

Rule 5 — Prioritize goals.

Some goals are more important than others. They must be prioritized on the basis of need, value, and time constraints. To help sort out each goal, classify them according to three categories: short, medium, and long-range.

Short-range goals are accomplished between today and the next several months. Deadlines are essential. Medium-range goals fall between one and several years. Both short and medium-range goals need to be very specific.

Long-range goals give overall direction and guidance and do not need to be as specific. An example of a long-range goal would be, "When I retire, I want to live near the coast with my family."

Medium and long-range goals are sustained and realized through the application of short-range goals.

What we do now determines what comes knocking at our door tomorrow. Our health is not an event where something is accomplished – it is a life-style. What we eat for breakfast, lunch and dinner, how we deal with stress, how often we exercise, and the level of our drinking all determine our health in the years to come.

Rule 6 — Goals must be written down.

The best way to anchor a goal is to write it down. There is something compelling about wet ink on dry paper. Goals that are not written down are easily forgotten. They have little chance of becoming anything more than great intentions.

Every goal should be outlined in small steps and presented in a realistic and achievable format. Planning to run a six-minute mile by the end of the week is an unrealistic goal if someone is out of physical condition. Radical change in a diet can also be a little shattering. Each of us is the best judge of our abilities and can best set our own goals. The object is to turn thought into action.

Rule 7 — Goals must have action behind them.

Once identified, we need to act on our goals immediately; it does not matter how much is done at first. What matters most is that people act swiftly. This might mean placing a telephone call or finding an old pair of running shoes. Digging the shoes out of the closet gets the ball rolling. Prevailing over any challenge starts with the smallest step.

If we find the shoes, put them on, and go for a walk, soon we will be running and will need new shoes.

> If we all did the things we are capable of doing, we would literally astound ourselves.
>
> — *Thomas A. Edison*

Rule 8 — Never give up.

The only time a goal should be abandoned is when that goal has been reevaluated and will no longer serve our best interest. If we really want something, we must put one foot in front of the other until we get there. Too many people give up just before their goals or dreams turn into reality. Keep in mind, if we give up, we will surely fail.

> Austere perseverance, harsh and continuous,
> may be employed by the smallest of us
> and rarely fails of its purpose,
> for its silent power
> grows irresistibly greater with time.
>
> —*Goethe*

Gout: *A metabolic disorder that leads to arthritic attacks of pain, inflammation, and swelling around joints.* High levels of uric acid, called *hyperuricemia*, are a major symptom of gout. It is not true that gout only affects the big toe.

MYTH

Excessive drinking causes gout.

REALITY

Although alcohol abuse tends to lead to hyperuricemia, it is generally accepted that alcoholics are no more prone to develop gout than nondrinkers. Alcohol can, however, aggravate gout. Light to moderate drinking is not recommended for those people with gouty arthritis.

Habits: *An acquired behavioral pattern developed and nurtured by repetition.* The addictive nature of alcohol can cause more than a habit, it can become a destructive addiction.

> We first make our habits,
> and then our habits make us.
>
> — *John Dryden*

Habits can be big or small, productive or unproductive, healthy or unhealthy, wanted or unwanted. Most of the time, we are not aware of the influence habits have on our lives. Regardless, we become more entrenched with habits as time passes.

> We are what we repeatedly do.
>
> — *Aristotle*

Repetition feeds habits. Just as they are learned, habits can be unlearned. We best manage habits by reinforcing healthy ones, and weeding out those that are unhealthy or unproductive.

Our personality and physical well-being are forged by the habits we collect. A drinking habit is nurtured when it is learned that alcohol fulfills a certain need. When a connection is made between alcohol and relaxation, a drinking habit may emerge if no further awareness or action is taken.

It is not simple to change old habits, beliefs, and

behaviors. Anything worth having is usually neither free nor easy, but the price of positive change is usually inconsequential relative to the rewards change brings.

Unlearning a drinking habit begins with the conscious thought that drinking brings more pain than pleasure. Then a decision is made to replace the practice of drinking with some other behavior. Extinguishing such a habit requires reinforcement, repetition, and time, much like the process that formed the habit.

> Habit is habit,
> and not to be flung out of the window
> by any man,
> but coaxed downstairs a step at a time.
>
> — *Mark Twain*

Regardless of the amount of time that passes, some folks will never change their behavior. For other people, habits can be changed in a few weeks. In many cases, simply developing an awareness that a habit exists is a tremendous leap forward.

Changing a drug habit is more challenging if it has developed into an addiction. A person may want to change, but the compulsion to continue drives them to repeat the behavior over and over.

Certain drugs produce such strong addictions that severe withdrawal symptoms can result when people try to end the addiction. Alcohol is one such commonly used drug.

Tips to break habits and make new ones

Many long-term habits, such as *wasting time*, have most likely consumed a large slice of some people's lives. Ending a time-consuming habit or changing a life-style can be an unbearable experience if new habits are not ready to replace old ones.

Be creative. Think of a habit that needs changing. If it is a drinking habit, think of things that could be substituted for drinking.

Breaking and Making Habits

Identify a habit that needs changing.

____

____

Question the habit. Does the habit serve a purpose anymore?

____

____

Identify what contributed to the formation of the habit. Was a drinking habit kindled by excess stress? What are the roots still feeding the habit?

____

____

____

____

Make sure the substitute habit is healthier than the habit being replaced. This is the whole point of changing habits. What are you going to do differently?

____

____

____

____

Habituation: *The process of developing a drinking habit or acquiring a tolerance to alcohol.* In either case, habituation signals trouble. This condition describes a person who has been drinking alcohol excessively over a period of time. It is wise to catch such a situation before it becomes a larger problem. Many folks need to be reminded that it is never too late to make changes that mark new directions.

> Ah, nothing is too late,
> Till the tired heart shall cease to palpitate.
>
> — *Longfellow*

Hangover: *A condition resulting in nausea, dizziness, vomiting, headaches, depression, and anxiety resulting from the consumption of too much alcohol.*

> A drunken night makes a cloudy morning.
>
> — *Sir William Cornwallis*

MYTH

Hangovers can be prevented
by drinking 100 percent pure alcohol.

REALITY

Hangovers are produced by a number of factors: lack of sleep, lowered blood sugar, withdrawal, congeners (impurities) and dehydration. To some degree, all contribute to the misery of the dreaded hangover blues. Any source of alcohol is the villain.

Drinking the next morning to "hold off" a hangover is an exercise in futility. It is not a remedy.

Although the exact cause of a hangover is not well understood, physical symptoms are well documented: headache, fatigue, upset stomach, thirst, depression, and general malaise. Their severity is determined by the quantity and type of alcohol consumed. The higher the blood alcohol level, the more likely a hangover will occur.

Congeners, or "impurities," present in alcoholic drinks contribute to hangovers. Red wines, brandy, and bourbon are examples of alcoholic drinks containing a high level of congeners. Vodka and many beers have much lower levels. Distilled spirits contain the highest levels, especially as they age.

Hangover symptoms can also be related to the body's withdrawal from alcohol and the dehydration caused by its diuretic effect. Physical and mental fatigue add to the general feeling of malaise.

Hard liquor: *Alcoholic beverages containing a high level of alcohol.* Rum, vodka, gin, and whisky are all examples of hard liquor. All contain approximately 40-50 percent alcohol (80 -100 proof).

Drinks containing hard liquor are often masked behind seemingly harmless names: "Fuzzy Bears," "Squirrels," "Watermelons," and "Long Island Tea." Behind the innocent facade is a half-ounce or more of a powerful drug called alcohol.

"Soft liquor," for lack of a better term, refers to alcoholic beverages that are lower in alcohol content. Although beer and wine fall into this category, they can be every bit as harmful as "hard liquor."

Health foods and drinks: *Foods and drinks that provide an abundance of essential nutrients without too many fats, sugars, and calories.*

For drinkers and nondrinkers alike, eating well is of vital importance. As conscientious consumers, we have the power to make sensible choices. Junk food can provide some basic nutrients, but the nutrients are overshadowed by the sugar and fat calories in the junk food.

Heart and artery disease: *An illness of the heart and accompanying arteries, or "fuel lines," that feed the heart.*

MYTH

Drinking is good for the heart.

REALITY

Few, if any, medical or health organizations encourage or support the use of alcohol to bolster the health of any organ in the body, let alone the heart. Any benefit from light to moderate drinking is usually overshadowed by the potential harm of drinking.

"Startling new discoveries" that sporadically make headlines can confuse people who become enlightened or disillusioned about what advice to follow. There have been thousands of research articles and books exposing the hazards of alcohol. Occasionally, a viewpoint emerges touting the health benefits of alcohol. View such information as a "red flag" signaling caution.

If a claim is proven valid, however, a medical and scientific consensus will emerge regarding recommendations for alcohol use in medicine.

It does not make good sense to risk other health problems by drinking alcohol just to possibly get a slight improvement in one area of our health.

If we look hard and long enough, something harmful can begin to look appealing when isolated and taken out of context.

> Although light to moderate drinking has been associated with decreased risk of coronary artery disease, the risk of arrhythmias (disruption of heart rhythm), cardiomyopathy (heart muscle disease), hypertension (high blood pressure), and hemorrhagic stroke increases significantly when alcohol is consumed on a regular basis beyond the moderate level.[23]

DID YOU KNOW?

If we have a normal heart, we probably do not think about it very often. Our hearts beat quietly and miraculously about 100,000 times per day. A healthy heart delivers an enormous volume of blood and nutrients throughout the body with great accuracy and precision. There has never been a "pump" more amazing or forgiving than the heart. Despite stress and poor dietary or exercise habits, it will beat about two and one-half billion times by the time a person is 65 years old.

If we value the health of our hearts, we can make choices that benefit our health without side effects and unnecessary risks. To begin with, we can play and exercise more, watch our diet, and reduce stress.

Heart muscle disease: *A sickness and weakness of the heart muscle caused by chronic abuse of alcohol.* Alcohol-related heart muscle disease, medically known as alcoholic cardiomyopathy, is seen in heavy drinkers.

Over a 10-year period, heavy abuse of alcohol will have a major effect on the heart's ability to pump blood. Symptoms include shortness of breath, fatigue, enlargement of the heart, chest pains, and significantly restricted cardiac output. If a person is experiencing any of these symptoms, a physician should be contacted immediately.

Humor: *Something absurd, amusing, or comical that makes people laugh or smile.*

> Laughter can relieve tension,
> soothe the pain of disappointment,
> and strengthen the spirit for
> the formidable tasks that always lie ahead.
>
> — *Dwight D. Eisenhower*

Humor has many hidden powers and can cut through years of pent-up stress. On the surface, it may seem to have little purpose. Quite the contrary!

Research shows that humor is an effective weapon against stress. Fewer things are as destructive to life as stress. In fact, there is growing evidence that most illnesses can be traced directly to a person's state of mind.

Altering one's mood with alcohol to make things *seem* humorous is not an effective means for coping with stress. Drinking only masks a stressful situation. (Refer to section on *stress* for more information.)

Hypertension: *A medical term for high blood pressure.* Hypertension is sometimes called the "silent killer" because people may be unaware of its presence.

MYTH

The relaxing effect of alcohol lowers blood pressure.

REALITY

Medical research shows a definite link between alcohol use and hypertension. Generally, the more one drinks, the greater the impact. A few drinks a day can elevate blood pressure; a drink or less a day does not appear to have an effect on elevating blood pressure.

The effects of alcohol on blood pressure appear to be reversible. Drinkers who stop consuming alcohol can expect a significant drop in both their diastolic and systolic pressure.

DID YOU KNOW?

The risk of hypertension is increased when one consumes as little as two to three drinks per day.[24,25]

Consuming five or more drinks a day can increase fourfold the risk of hemorrhagic stroke.[26]

DID YOU KNOW?

The heart is composed of the *right* and *left* pump. Each pump has an atrium and ventricle. The blood returning from different parts of the body enters the right atrium of the heart via the inferior and superior vena cava. From the right atrium, the blood is pumped into the right ventricle. At the correct moment, the right ventricle contracts and the blood is pumped to the lungs via the pulmonary artery. This period is known as ***systole,*** the higher of the two numbers measuring a person's blood pressure.

After the blood has been oxygenated and disposed of carbon dioxide, it is returned to the left atrium of the heart. It then enters the left ventricle. Contraction of the left ventricle pumps the oxygenated blood into the systemic circulation via the aorta.

When the ventricles are filling with blood, the heart is in ***diastole,*** a relaxed state. This is reflected in the lower number when a person's blood pressure is taken.

Hypoglycemia: *"Reactive" hypoglycemia is a disorder marked by low blood sugar as a result of producing too much insulin after eating.* Insulin is responsible for moving blood sugar into billions of hungry body cells.

Hypoglycemics experience low blood sugar levels after eating sugary type foods that cause the release of too much insulin. Too much insulin release leads to less sugar in the blood.

The sugar in blood functions like gasoline in a fuel line that supplies energy to a car engine. A drop in the level of sugar can produce muscle weakness, hunger, sweating, dizziness, trembling, headache or confusion, all of which make for an unpleasant experience.

It is important to maintain appropriate levels of sugar in the blood, especially when exercising or not eating. Normally, to meet its energy needs, a body first draws from its special carbohydrate stores. Think of carbohydrates as fuel. Since the available sugar in these energy stores is quite limited, it is vital that the body be able to manufacture and process sugar to maintain a balance.

DID YOU KNOW?

People who are prone to hypoglycemia should refrain from drinking alcohol. They should also watch their intake of "sweets," and if required, seek professional advice on nutritional information for special diets.

Alcohol interferes with the body's natural ability to make sugar from body proteins when we do not eat sufficient food. This can cause the sugar level to drop. Since alcohol cannot be chemically changed to sugar, it also offers no help in sustaining normal blood sugar levels.

The use of alcohol and oral hypoglycemic drugs such as chlorpropamide can result in disulfiram-like reactions.[27]

Illicit drugs: *Drugs that are illegal to use or possess.* The term "controlled substance" is the preferred legal term for an illicit drug.

Immune system: *An organization of cells and proteins that defends the body from "bugs" or "foreign invaders."*

DID YOU KNOW?

> It is well documented from scientific studies that alcohol depresses the immune system.[28]

Potentially harmful organisms surround us in the form of viruses, bacteria, and fungi. They are invisible to the naked eye, and can hide in just about every crack and crevice we can see or touch. These invaders make their presence known by doing everything from rotting food to causing serious and fatal body infections.

Most of us rely, moment to moment, on our immune defense system to thwart the relentless attack of these deadly organisms. Defeating these organisms is the primary responsibility of a tenacious immune system.

Aside from the protection offered by our skin, the immune system has two major lines of defense working together to protect the body against infections. They are known as "B-lymphocytes" and "T-lymphocytes." Both are white blood cells that, as a team, mount a staggering defense on our behalf.

Unfortunately, alcohol abuse is known to suppress both B and T-lymphocyte systems. The immune system can become less protective as a person consumes greater amounts of alcohol. This gives viruses and bacteria that live within arm's reach a better chance to strike.

The immune system can also be suppressed by other factors such as poor dietary habits, inadequate rest, and stressful living.

Tips to Bolster the Immune System

- Eat nutritious foods on a regular basis.
- Get plenty of rest and adequate sleep.
- Stay physically fit by exercising regularly.
- Quit or reduce the level of alcohol consumption. As little as a few beers a day, or their equivalent, may temporarily dampen immune response.
- Keep a sense of humor. Humor has been known for years to diffuse stressful situations. When under stress, the body responds by releasing two hormones: epinephrine and cortisol.

  Both hormones and alcohol are known to increase blood pressure. Cortisol and alcohol, whether working together or alone, can significantly suppress the immune system.
- Ask a doctor about getting immunized against certain infectious diseases.

DID YOU KNOW?

> Drinking alcohol during pregnancy can compromise the immune system and may also increase the susceptibility of the newborn child to infectious diseases and cancer.[29]

Inebriety: *Excessive drinking to the point of intoxication.* (Refer to section on *intoxication.*)

Intervention: *Action steps taken to confront or interrupt an alcoholic's drinking behavior.*

MYTH

Forcing someone to acknowledge a drinking problem is the first step in the "enlightenment" process.

REALITY

Many people find any form of change to be uncomfortable and frightening. They resist being told or *advised* to do something different, especially when it comes to breaking old habits and facing sensitive issues. With encouragement and support, however, people have a way of changing.

> People have a way of becoming
> what you encourage them to be —
> not what you nag them to be.
>
> — Scudder N. Parker

Demanding or nagging an alcoholic to immediately face a drinking problem could prove counterproductive. Intense feelings of anxiety may result and actually encourage continued drinking. Gentle, but strong and steady family support, mixed with professional therapy, can provide a solid foundation for positive change. (Refer to section on *treatment*.)

Intoxication: *A condition brought about by drinking alcohol to the point of causing significant impairment of normal functions.*

DID YOU KNOW?

> It is the quantity of alcohol consumed, not the act of mixing alcoholic drinks, that leads to intoxication.

To more accurately define intoxication, the American Psychiatric Association has outlined specific criteria in the *Diagnostic and Statistical Manual DSM-IV* to diagnose Alcohol Intoxication:

Diagnostic Criteria for Alcohol Intoxication

The American Psychiatric Association's Diagnostic and Statistical Manual *DSM-IV* outlines criteria used to diagnose Alcohol Intoxication.

Group A response:

- ☐ Recent consumption of alcohol.

Group B response:

- ☐ Clinically significant behavioral or psychological changes that result during or shortly after alcohol has been ingested.

  – inappropriate or aggressive behavior
  – inappropriate sexual conduct
  – impaired judgment

Group C response:

- ☐ One or more of the following manifestations result during or shortly after alcohol has been ingested:

  – coma or stupor
  – impaired memory or attention
  – incoordination
  – nystagmus (involuntary eye movement)
  – slurred speech
  – unsteady gait (walking or stepping)

Group D response:

- ☐ The symptoms above are not a result of an existing medical condition or another mental disorder.

Note: Criteria A-D are essential features of alcohol intoxication. The degree of alcohol intoxication is related to the severity of symptoms.

Legal intoxication: *The blood alcohol level used to identify a person who is at risk or likely to receive a DUI (driving under the influence) citation.*

Legal intoxication levels may vary slightly from state to state. Check with current laws and regulations regarding specific states.

Life-style: *How we live day to day.*

> Your life is an expression of all your thoughts.
>
> — *Marcus Aurelius*

Before people can make changes in their daily living, they need to define what they like and dislike. It is important to make choices that support the change. The next table can be used as a guide toward changing life-styles:

Potential Life-style Changes

- ☐ Quit or decrease level of drinking
- ☐ Reduce level of stress
- ☐ Overcome certain fears that hold a person back
- ☐ Improve general level of health
- ☐ Improve diet and nutritional habits
- ☐ Increase general level of physical fitness
- ☐ Change body weight
- ☐ Improve physical appearance (shape)
- ☐ Be more adventurous
- ☐ Develop a more favorable image
- ☐ Have more fun each day
- ☐ Worry less
- ☐ Improve financial status
- ☐ Develop more personal friendships
- ☐ Change career or work responsibilities
- ☐ Have more spare time
- ☐ Travel more often
- ☐ Improve social standing in the community
- ☐ Be more confident and self-assured
- ☐ Waste less time
- ☐ Be more creative
- ☐ Accept oneself a little more
- ☐ Revamp or revise entire life-style
- ☐ Other . . . ________________________________

Light beer: *Beer that contains about 25 to 30 percent fewer calories, and sometimes up to 10 percent less alcohol, than regular beer.*

Lipoproteins and blood fats: *Special compounds found in the blood system that transport fats and cholesterol to various destinations in the body.*

Sometimes we think of blood fats as "artery cloggers." All too often people increase the risk of heart disease by eating too many rich fatty foods. "Rich and creamy" blood is the result of devouring too much fat. These blood fats need help to maneuver through the blood.

Various "transport vehicles," called lipoproteins, are specifically chartered to shuttle fats and cholesterol around in the blood. The type and number of these transporters can be used to determine the risk of developing heart disease.

Lipoproteins have been given nicknames by biochemists and doctors. HDLs (high density lipoproteins) and LDLs (low density lipoproteins) are two lipoproteins frequently discussed in connection with the risk of developing heart disease. HDLs are referred to as "good" cholesterol and LDLs are referred to as "bad" cholesterol.

For years, doctors have known that a high LDL count indicates an increased risk of heart disease. HDLs, in greater quantities, seem to significantly reduce that risk.

DID YOU KNOW?

In some individuals, light to moderate alcohol intake is thought to increase the level of HDLs. In many cases, this "bright side" to alcohol can lose its shine with time. If alcohol consumption increases and continues, alcohol's harmful effects outweigh any possible gain from lipoprotein changes.

People predisposed to elevated blood fats (medically known as *type IV hyperlipoproteinemia*) will find no comfort knowing that alcohol aggravates the condition.

Whether people drink or not, it is extremely important to watch their fat intake. Decreasing fat in one's diet is thought to increase one's life span.

How much is a good thing?

A screening can be performed to determine total cholesterol level in the blood. The total cholesterol represents all the cholesterol found in blood lipoproteins. A reading of less than 200 is favorable. A number significantly below 200 is even better.

Cholesterol levels between 200 and 239 are considered "borderline-high," and are a signal to start modifying one's diet. A level of 240 or above indicates a cholesterol problem that needs immediate attention.

A lower risk of heart disease exists if:

- HDL cholesterol level above 60
- LDL cholesterol below 130

A higher risk of heart disease exists if:

- HDL cholesterol below 35
- LDL cholesterol-159 (borderline high)
- LDL cholesterol above 160 (high)
- Total cholesterol to HDL above 4.5
- Ratio of LDL to HDL is greater than 5 to 1

Keep in mind, we do not need cholesterol in our diets. Our bodies manufacture sufficient amounts to meet our daily needs.

Where Are the Fats in Foods?

Butter • vegetable oils • margarine
mayonnaise • salad oils • shortening

100 %

Cheese • bacon • bologna • avocados • olives,
peanut butter • sour cream • nuts • beef franks

70-80+ %

Hamburgers • french fries • ice cream • medium-fat meat
whole milk • chocolate bars • fried chicken • potato chips

50-60+ %

2% low-fat milk • cupcakes • biscuits • cookies
salmon • lean-meat • dark turkey (w/o skin)

30-40+ %

Plain low-fat yogurt • 1% low-fat milk
oysters • light turkey (w/o skin)

20-30+%

Most kinds of bread • hamburger buns • plain pancakes

10-20+%

Beans • shrimp • lobster • cod • clams
most breakfast cereals • English muffins

5-10+%

Fruit • skim milk • sugar • rice • colas • popcorn
• spaghetti • most vegetables • bulgur • pasta

0-5+%

Liquors: *Alcoholic drinks made from distilled spirits, various flavorings, and sweeteners.* The alcohol content is usually between 18 and 30 percent. Many people treat these drinks as though they were hors d'oeuvres or desserts, forgetting each one is loaded with alcohol.

Liver disease: *An unhealthy condition of the liver that interferes or prevents it from performing normal functions.* Alcohol abuse is a common cause of liver disease.

The liver is one of the busiest organs in the body, and performs a number of incredible feats every minute. Aside from being the major theater for drug metabolism, the liver stores certain nutrients, manufactures essential compounds, destroys unneeded materials, and regulates countless metabolic reactions.

MYTH

Liver disease is irreversible.

REALITY

In many cases, the body can recover from short-term alcohol abuse; there are, however, limits. Chronic or sustained alcohol abuse will eventually take its toll. There is good news for people who stop drinking: various liver diseases, short of cirrhosis, are thought to be somewhat reversible.

Chronic alcohol abuse can lead to three different liver diseases: fatty liver, alcoholic hepatitis, and cirrhosis.

Fatty liver

The first stage of liver disease occurs with fat accumulation in the liver. Normally, the liver makes fat and ships it to the blood for deposit in fat storage sites.

Alcohol encourages the development of fatty liver by increasing fat production and slowing the movement of fat out of the liver.

By reducing or abstaining from alcohol, the liver can clear itself of fat. A well-balanced, nutritious diet will also help nurture the liver and restore its health.

Alcoholic hepatitis

Alcoholic hepatitis is a liver disease characterized by inflammation and liver necrosis (death of tissue cells). It appears in alcoholics or heavy drinkers after a severe or prolonged period of excessive drinking. Some major symptoms in mild alcoholic hepatitis include: jaundice (yellow tainting of the skin and white part of the eyes), anorexia (loss of appetite), fatigue, intermittent low-grade fever, occasional nausea and vomiting, and a general feeling of weakness and ill health. Alcoholic hepatitis can be reversed if a person abstains from drinking.

Cirrhosis

Cirrhosis is a very serious condition. It is characterized by the widespread loss of healthy liver cells that have been replaced with nonfunctional scar tissue. These bands of fibrous scar tissue reduce the blood supply to the liver cells. Eventually, these cells are unable to perform.

After the liver loses its ability to effectively remove toxic substances, the buildup of poisons can cause problems as these toxins circulate in the blood. Mental confusion and impaired memory are two symptoms of toxic substances in the brain.

Poor blood circulation is another serious problem caused by a diseased liver. After blood is pumped throughout the body to supply oxygen and nutrients to cells, it passes through the liver on its journey back to the heart. Impaired blood flow throughout the liver can increase pressure in certain blood vessels. This can lead to distended blood vessels in the esophagus and other organs. If the vessels continue to enlarge, they may rupture and cause hemorrhaging.

Although advanced stages of liver disease and cirrhosis are generally irreversible, it is never too late to seek medical advice and treatment.

Cirrhosis of the liver usually occurs after many years of alcohol abuse. Cirrhosis is more likely to develop, however, in people who drink 80 grams of alcohol per day for more than 10 years. Eighty grams of alcohol is the equivalent of a six-pack of 12-ounce beers. This dose may be significantly lower or higher for some people; no specific measurement of alcohol consumption can determine the development of cirrhosis.

DID YOU KNOW?

It has been estimated that the life expectancy of a person afflicted by alcoholic liver disease is shortened between nine and 22 years.[30]

Malnutrition: *The result of consuming food that fails the body's nutritional needs.*

Drinking too much alcohol is a major contributing factor for malnutrition. Alcoholics are malnourished for several reasons. First, alcohol replaces nutritious foods in the diet. Alcoholic beverages are notorious for being sources of "empty calories." For instance, 20 ounces of 86 proof liquor provides approximately 1,500 kcals (about one-half to two-thirds of a person's daily energy requirement) without providing significant amounts of protein, vitamins, or minerals.

Alcohol can cause inflammation of the stomach, pancreas, and intestine, which can result in malabsorption of nutrients. Two notable examples are thiamine and folacin, both important B complex vitamins. Further deficiencies occur when the kidneys are forced by alcohol to increase the excretion of certain nutrients, such as magnesium, zinc, and potassium.

The metabolite acetaldehyde, which is formed when alcohol is initially broken down, can interfere with the activation of some vitamins in the liver. Several selected vitamins must be activated or converted into a usable form before they can function in the body. Depressed levels of active vitamin D, pyridoxine, and thiamin are found in some alcoholics.

Overall, diminished nutrient availability can also be attributed to depressed food intake. Hunger and appetite depend to some extent on the amount of alcohol ingested. Light consumption can stimulate appetite, while excessive use tends to curb interest in food.

Malt liquor: *An alcoholic drink resembling beer.* The alcohol content is between 6.5 and 7 percent.

Marijuana: *A preparation of leafy material derived from cannabis plants.* Marijuana, one of the most prevalent illegal drugs used in the United States, continues to cause major concerns and problems in our society. The potency of marijuana's physiological effect is directly related to the quantity of the active mind altering substance known as delta-9 tetrahydrocannabinol (THC) found in the stems and leaves of cannabis plants. Although hundreds of chemical substances are produced from burning marijuana, THC is the primary psychoactive substance obtained from eating or smoking marijuana.

MYTH

Marijuana is not addictive.

REALITY

According to the American Psychiatric Association's *Diagnostic and Statistical Manual* (*DSM-IV*), compulsive use of marijuana can lead to chemical dependency.

DID YOU KNOW?

Marijuana use is linked to lung cancer, emphysema, bronchitis, decreased pulmonary or lung function, short-term memory loss, short- and long-term cognitive impairment, poor concentration and interference with learning, visual distortions, depressed motor or physical activity, reproductive disorders, tachycardia, suppressed immune response, and anxiety. In many cases marijuana produces hallucinations, panic attacks, paranoia, and the curiosity to potentially experiment with other drugs.

Memory: *The ability to retain and recall previously learned information.* All of us wish we had more *memory* when trying to recall a name, date, or place when it is stubbornly lodged on the tip of our tongue.

Calling upon our memory is a complex process. Let's simplify the mechanics of it. The brain's first job starts when it receives facts and encodes information. After the information is deciphered, it must be translated or consolidated into a form that can be stored in the brain. To use or recall "memory," stored information must be retrieved from numerous storage sites.

MYTH

Heavy drinking has little impact on memory.

REALITY

Chronic or excessive drinking can devastate a person's memory. Both short-term and long-term memory can be affected. Most experts believe that alcohol damages memory by interfering with the encoding of information. It is as if thoughts were never recorded in the brain. The result is simple: less thoughts can be retrieved when less information is stored.

A blood alcohol level as low as the legal limit for driving may subtly affect the brain's ability to handle information. As the blood alcohol level increases, memory impairment increases. The results become quite noticeable after years of heavy drinking.

Memory tolerance: *The body's ability to remember that the body had earlier developed a tolerance to alcohol.*

A person who develops a tolerance to alcohol requires more alcohol to elicit the same physiological effect on the mind and body that once required less alcohol.

Continuous drug use means a greater tolerance to alcohol. The body tissues become less sensitive to the drug or the liver becomes more efficient in degrading the drug.

After people establish a tolerance to alcohol, they develop a "memory tolerance." In other words, that tolerance is not easily forgotten by the body. Should they resume drinking after a period of sobriety, their bodies adjust quickly to their former tolerance to alcohol.

Metabolic tolerance: *An increased ability to metabolize a drug.* The body, like the mind, can take just so much "bashing" by drugs before mounting a defense against further attacks.

The responsibilities of the liver are so great that it cannot allow alcohol to trample its important metabolic functions. Consequently, the liver defends itself by increasing the rate of destroying alcohol.

DID YOU KNOW?

Heavy long-term drinking weakens and erodes tolerance. The protective defense against excessive intake of alcohol can crumble into ruin with more advanced drinking habits.

Mistakes: *Errors in judgment or performance.* In the "old days," mistakes were called blunders, foul-ups, or goofs. All of us have made them. Wise people realize that mistakes are opportunities for learning.

Most of us were taught that mistakes should be avoided, as if they were not a natural part of life. Yet people who have succeeded have a history of mistakes riddled with failures. The key point to learn from making mistakes is to turn them into valuable lessons.

People grow by solving problems, not by drinking to cope with mistakes. If they choose to drink, problems magnify and mistakes can increase.

> The man who does things makes many mistakes, but he never makes the biggest mistake of all — doing nothing.
>
> — *Benjamin Franklin*

Motivation: *A prompting or encouragement to act; the coming together of motive and action.*

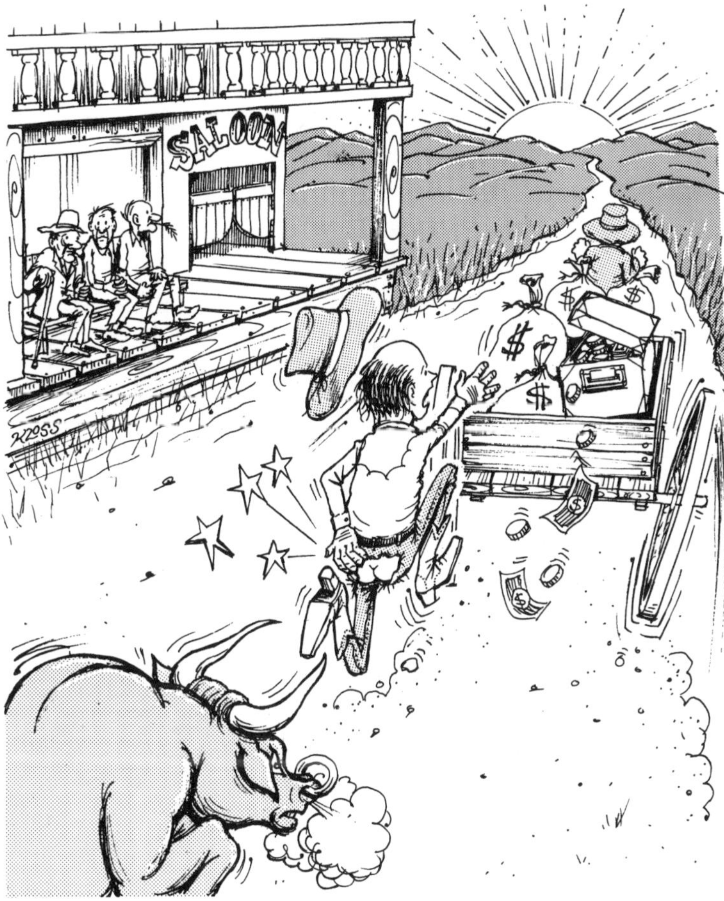

Need a little motivation?

Motivation is a "push and pull" phenomenon. Each of us is pushed or nudged by inherent desires and needs — food, health, love, and security being the most basic needs. By the same token, we are pulled along by rewards and incentives — money and success being powerful motivators. To stay motivated a person needs to be pushed and pulled. People can be driven to want something, but without an incentive, motivation eventually fades.

Motivation, by its very nature, has many interesting facets. A person, for example, who overeats to satisfy a ravenous appetite for food is highly motivated by the pleasures that delicious foods provide. Similarly, stress is a powerful motivator prompting people to seek comfort in drinking, overeating, and participating in other unhealthy life-style habits. Until healthy alternatives are considered to handle stress, relief and peace-of-mind will remain elusive. On the other hand, a person who has made a firm commitment to change their life-style and learn how to deal with stress can be equally motivated. This is a classic example of two motivated individuals heading in two entirely different directions.

The Key to Motivation

The motivation to change habits depends on understanding how a desire or need impacts our decisions. A *desire* is nothing more than an interest in something. When a desire occupies your thoughts on a regular basis, driving you to take action, the process for change has begun. A *need* is a more intense, compelling motivator requiring immediate attention. If a physical or emotional need is not satisfied, the consequences can be intolerable or unacceptable. The motivation required to change behavior and life-style habits is found in our *need* to avoid pain and seek pleasure and rewards.

If people want to change their drinking habits, they need to believe that the physical, mental, and emotional rewards of not drinking outweigh any temporary effects of alcohol. This type of "pull" helps people stay motivated.

Mouthwash: *An oral disinfectant used for killing bacteria and refreshing the mouth.*

DID YOU KNOW?

> Many mouthwashes contain alcohol. Read the labels before choosing one. Some brands have a 20 percent alcohol content.

Narcotic: *A "controlled substance" drug that has painkilling properties and resembles an opiate, such as morphine and codeine.*

The danger of mixing alcohol with narcotic drugs cannot be overstated. Heed the warning advice on labels or packaged instructions when taking prescribed narcotic medications.

Nonalcoholic beer: *Beers with alcohol removed.*

MYTH

Nonalcoholic beers are alcohol-free.

REALITY

In the strictest sense, nonalcoholic beers are not completely alcohol-free. They actually contain less than 0.5 percent alcohol. This means one 12-ounce nonalcoholic beer contains about one gram of alcohol. If someone drank a six-pack of nonalcoholic beer, they would have consumed approximately six grams of alcohol. Arguably, this is a slight amount, given most regular 12-ounce beers contain about 13 grams of alcohol.

Nutrients: *Chemical substances found in food that sustain the body.* They provide energy and materials for growth and nourishment to cells throughout the body.

DID YOU KNOW?

> Alcohol can rob the body of important vitamins, minerals, and water.

Many unsuspecting drinkers rob themselves of important nutrients. Heavy drinkers receive a large portion of their energy needs from alcohol, not from nutritious foods. Alcohol interferes with the absorption and retention of some important nutrients. As time passes, deficiencies of essential nutrients become commonplace.

Essential nutrients must be consumed through the diet

since the body does not manufacture them. The six nutrient groups are: carbohydrates (sugars and starches), lipids (fats), proteins, vitamins, minerals, and water.

Carbohydrate, fat, and protein are the three fuel nutrients burned by the body to provide energy. Although alcohol is a rich source of energy, it is considered a toxic nutrient and has no place among the essential nutrients.

Although we obtain zero energy from vitamins, minerals, and water, certain vitamins and minerals act like spark plugs, setting energy-producing nutrients on fire.

Vitamins and minerals do much more than burn fuels. Let's take a quick glance at them. As *organic* nutrients, vitamins are required in very small quantities in the diet. They perform many vital functions that contribute to the release of energy from food. Other general functions include their involvement in reproduction, vision, bone development, and blood formation and clotting.

Minerals are special types of *inorganic* nutrients. They are also required in very small quantities for the purpose of serving the needs of billions of body cells. Those functions include: growth and repair of body tissues, transmission of nerve impulses, regulation of muscle contraction, maintenance of water balance, and structural roles.

Water is an important lubricant. It also works to cool and maintain normal cell operation. Alcohol tends to rob the body of this much needed nutrient. When too much water is excreted, *dehydration* results.

The following table is a list of all the essential nutrients our bodies need:

Essential Nutrients

Carbohydrates

Lipids

linoleic acid and linolenic acid

Proteins

Essential amino acids

leucine
isoleucine
lysine
methionine
phenylalanine
threonine
tryptophan
valine
histidine

Vitamins

Fat-soluble

A (retinol)
E (tocopherol)
D (cholecalciferol)
K (quinones)

Water-soluble

thiamine (B1)
riboflavin (B2)
niacin
pyridoxine (B6)
ascorbic acid (C)
biotin
pantothenic acid
cobalamin (B12)
folacin

Minerals

Macronutrients

calcium
phosphorus
potassium
sulfur
sodium
chloride
magnesium

Micronutrients

iron
manganese
copper
iodine
chromium
molybdenum
cobalt
fluorine
selenium
zinc

Water

Nutrition: *The science or study of food.* Good nutrition begins with eating nutritious foods to promote and sustain health.

MYTH

A nutritious diet will protect drinkers
from alcohol-related health problems.

REALITY

It is not news that a well-balanced diet is preferred over a poor diet. Many major medical problems evident in people abusing alcohol are compounded by poor nutritional habits. Although drinkers benefit from eating healthy foods, there are no assurances that a good diet will spare them from liver disease or other ailments. Alcoholics who "drink" their meals from a bottle are poorly nourished.

The choices and decisions made daily about what types of food to eat will have a tremendous impact on an individual's health and vitality. Food is much more than a source of energy. Eating a variety of nutritious foods will adequately provide the essential nutrients a person needs on a regular basis.

Nutritional value of alcoholic beverages: *The nutritional density of particular foods or beverages.* It is determined by the ratio of nutrients to calories. A food or drink that is low in calories and high in nutrients is a high-quality, nutrient-dense substance.

MYTH

Alcoholic drinks are a good source for certain nutrients.

REALITY

It depends on how the drinks are made. Beer, wine, and distilled drinks should never be considered a significant source of nutrients. Glance at the next table to quiet any doubts.

Trying to redeem the nutritional value of a hard drink with tomato juice or orange juice, or with a slice of pineapple seems a bit ridiculous. But, in these instances, one would have to agree with the old adage, "Something is better than nothing."

How Nutritious are Alcoholic Drinks?

A person would have to consume the following number of drinks every day to satisfy the need for the following nutrients for only one day!

Beer (12-ounce cans/day)	Wine (3.5-ounce glasses/day)
10 - 20 cans magnesium • riboflavin	**20 - 40 glasses** iron • magnesium
40 - 60 cans thiamine • calcium protein	**40 - 60 glasses** riboflavin
80 - 120 cans iron • niacin	**100 - 150 glasses** zinc • calcium
130 - 170 cans zinc	**180 - 350 glasses** niacin • thiamine protein

Distilled spirits provide virtually zero nutrition. Beer, wine, and distilled spirits are not a significant source of nutrients.

One fluid ounce of alcohol: *One fluid ounce of alcohol is equal to approximately 23 grams of pure alcohol, or the equivalent of two 12-ounce beers.* People who consume an average of one or more ounces of alcohol a day are considered heavy drinkers.

Osteoporosis: *A "porous bone" disease characterized by decreased bone density without a change in the bone's chemical composition.* An easy way to picture this condition is to visualize the effect of drilling holes through a block of wood. The wood surrounding the holes remains untouched. The block of wood, however, becomes more porous and weaker as each hole is drilled.

The bones that make up the human skeleton develop throughout childhood. They tend to reach their peak bone mass and strength in late adolescence or the early twenties.

The principal determinant for adult bone strength depends on the bone mass accumulated during the "growing" years and on the amount lost with age.

Osteoporosis accounts for many of the bone fractures seen in aging people. As a person becomes older, the risk of suffering from bone fractures increases. Approximately 25 million people in the United States, mostly older women, suffer from this condition. This is especially true for menopausal women and for people with a history of drinking.

DID YOU KNOW?

Heavy alcohol use accelerates the demineralization process called "thinning of bones." Alcohol is believed to decrease the absorption of calcium present in food and to increase the excretion of calcium from the body. Problems develop when more calcium leaves the body than comes in. Both men and women are at risk of bone loss from drinking and from not having well-balanced diets.

Risk Factors Associated With Bone Loss

- Heavy alcohol use
- Menopause
- Amenorrhea (lack of menstrual periods)
- Physical inactivity
- Age
- Gender (being a female)
- Low calcium intake
- High protein diets
- Low body weight
- Excessive caffeine use
- Glucocorticoid use
- High fiber intake
- Cigarette smoking

Prevention of bone-related diseases focuses on two major strategies: optimizing peak bone mass during the formative years, and reducing age-related or life-style-related bone loss. Remember, an unhealthy life-style cannot be cured by swallowing a pill or by taking a supplement. The following table shows ways to reduce the risk of developing weak bones:

How to Reduce the Risk of Developing Weak Bones

- Develop a life-style that supports routine exercise. This is good for the heart and bones, and a great way of reducing and coping with stress in life.

  Alcohol and stress accentuate the release of adrenal corticoids hormones (stress hormones) that tend to lead to bone loss.

- Develop a good sense for foods. Consuming a variety of nutritious foods daily that supply the 40 plus essential nutrients is critical to develop and maintain the health of all body tissues.

  Meeting the recommendation (RDA) for calcium is especially important for individuals who are potential candidates of bone-related diseases. The RDA for calcium for both males and females between the ages of 11 and 24 is 1,200 mg per day. For most other people the RDA is 800 mg per day.

- Avoid smoking and drinking alcohol. Alcohol can affect judgment, so undemanding physical activities can become potentially dangerous.

- Shortly before menopause, women should discuss the risks and benefits of estrogen replacement therapy with their physician. It is also important to discuss healthy life-style choices and habits.

Patience: *A wonderful blend of perseverance and composure.*

> The heights by great men reached and kept
> were not attained by sudden flight, but they,
> while their companions slept,
> were toiling upward in the night.
>
> — Henry Wadsworth Longfellow

Expecting habits to suddenly disappear is an experience in frustration. We owe it to ourselves to be patient with changes.

Physical dependence: *A key symptom characterizing an addiction to a drug.* Physical dependence is characterized by increased tolerance. Withdrawal symptoms can occur if the person restricts the amount of the drug consumed. (Refer to section on *alcohol dependence*.)

Physical fitness: *The condition of the body that determines its ability to perform various physical activities.* For many years, *physical fitness* referred to a person's capacity for movement. In the narrowest sense, physical fitness relates to a person's ability to maneuver and compete in a variety of athletic events.

More recently, people in the wellness field are concentrating on the relationship between physical fitness and health. The term *health-related physical fitness* is used more often to stress the importance of physical activity to enhance health, endurance, strength, flexibility, longevity, and to decrease the risk of disease, disability, and premature death.

For most of us, the goal of physical fitness does not include running the fastest race or hitting the most baseballs in a season. It does, however, mean developing and maintaining a life-style with activities that promote health, happiness, and a positive attitude.

One enormous benefit of physical fitness is the positive impact it has on improving a person's attitude and self-esteem. Masking a poor self-image with alcohol abuse is no match for the uplifting benefits of exercise.

> Those who think they have not time
> for bodily exercise will sooner or later
> have to find time for illness.
>
> *— Edward Stanley, 15th Earl of Derby*

Problems: *Challenges that require solutions.* Problems come in different sizes and shapes. They are also given different names. Some people refer to them as obstacles. Other people may call them hassles, dilemmas, predicaments, or just irritations.

Problems cannot be solved until we understand their roots. Answers are found by analyzing problems. For every answer, there is a preexisting question, and for every solution, there was once a problem.

> Every problem contains within itself
> the seeds of its own solution.
>
> — Stanley Arnold

The person with a drinking problem has a specific set of problems. Despite the type or magnitude of their problems, it is important that they confront them honestly. The nature of a problem is secondary to how it is handled.

> It is in the whole process
> of meeting and solving problems
> that life has meaning.
> Problems are the cutting edge
> that distinguishes
> between success and failure.
> Problems call forth our courage and our wisdom;
> indeed, they create our courage and wisdom.
> It is only because of problems that we grow
> mentally and spiritually.
> It is through the pain
> of confronting and resolving problems
> that we learn.
>
> — Scott Peck

Proof: *A method of identifying the amount of alcohol in distilled liquor.* The percentage of pure alcohol in liquor is determined by dividing the proof number by two. For instance, 80 proof alcohol is 40 percent alcohol.

Proteins: *One of the six major nutrient groups essential to a balanced diet.* The word "protein" causes many people to think of meat, milk, cheese, and eggs. Health experts realize that proteins found in cereals, beans, and many other plant products, contribute enough protein to the diet without the need for such animal products.

Regardless of the source, all proteins are quickly broken down into "building blocks" called amino acids. They are eventually used for tissue building and repair, and are also a potential source of energy.

Individuals who *drink* a portion of their meals should pay close attention. Typically, about 10 percent of total caloric intake should come from protein. For the average woman or man, this amounts to 50 and 60 grams of protein a day respectively.

"Essential" and "nonessential" amino acids are the two kinds of amino acids found in proteins. The term *essential* refers to what the body cannot make and must be consumed through the diet. *Nonessential* amino acids are easily produced in a healthy body.

Satisfying the need for essential amino acids can be accomplished by consuming proteins from animal sources, called “complete” proteins. It can also be satisfied by eating a variety of plant protein foods, containing the "incomplete" proteins. Proteins found in animal tissue are considered "complete" high quality proteins. They contain all of the necessary essential amino acids the body needs. Incomplete proteins found in plants are often referred to as lower quality proteins, as they are deficient in one or more essential amino acids.

The fact that individual plant proteins such as rice and beans lack all the required essential amino acids is not a problem. It is irrelevant that amino acids come from plant or animal tissue as long as all the essential amino acid needs are satisfied.

Consider combining cereals and beans. Cereals are low in one type of essential amino acid (lysine); beans are low in another essential amino acid (methionine). If we eat both of these foods together, each food complements the other, so neither lysine nor methionine are missing from the diet.

Psychoactive drugs: *Drugs that alter biochemical functions of the brain that cause changes in thought, consciousness, emotions, and behavior.*

Common Psychoactive Drugs

Stimulants:
- Amphetamines, cocaine, caffeine (mild)

Depressants:
- Alcohol, barbiturates, benzodiazepines, hypnotics, sedatives

Narcotics:
- Opium, heroin, morphine, codeine, methadone

Hallucinogens:
- LSD, psilocybin, mescaline, PCP, peyote

Cannabis:
- Marijuana, hashish, tetrahydrocannabinol

Psychotherapeutic:
- Drugs prescribed by physicians to treat mental disorders.

Relaxation: *A self-induced, stress-free state of mind and body.* People who drink are encouraged to relax naturally. The following exercise may be helpful for anyone seeking a stress-free moment:

Find a comfortable place on the floor to relax. The back must be completely flat with the lower portion pressed gently against the floor. A small pillow or towel placed under the knees will help support the lower back. Arms and legs should be slightly spread apart.

Enjoy the comfort of the room. Breathe gently. Slow, deep rhythmic breathing calms the body more quickly and effectively than any other known relaxation technique.

Feel the body weight being supported by the floor. Rest and continue to breathe. Let the eyes close. Each full breath of air nourishes the blood and soothes the body. Slowly exhale.

The brain shifts to different kinds of electrical wave patterns when the body is relaxed. In deepened relaxed states, more alpha waves (associated with calmness, harmony, creativity, and well-being) are produced.

Simple Tips for Relaxation

- Take walks
- Stretch
- Develop hobbies
- Find activities that give pleasure
- Meditate
- Take little naps now and then
- Develop close friendships with positive people
- Sing or listen to music
- Listen to trees rustle in the breeze
- Breathe deeply from the diaphragm
- Play games
- Practice positive affirmations and thinking
- Improve eating habits
- Daydream
- Take a hot bath or shower

Remission: *The pause, interruption, or abstention from drinking.* The word *remission* is sometimes used to describe recovery for alcoholics who have stopped drinking.

It is thought that there is an increased likelihood for former alcoholics to resume uncontrolled drinking if they start drinking any amount of alcohol. Although this position has been challenged, using any alcohol or engaging in activities that encourage old drinking habits is not recommended.

DID YOU KNOW?

> A relapse, or return to drinking, can occur for a number of reasons: inability to cope with stress, anxiety, depression, the availability of alcohol, personal problems, social pressures, genetic and/or physiological differences.

Resources: *A source of information or service providing assistance to people with questions about particular subjects.* A person's greatest strength can be found in seeking help from other people.

> The greatest genius will not be worth much
> if he pretends to draw exclusively
> from his own resources.
>
> — Goethe

Invaluable information is just a postage stamp, email or telephone call away:

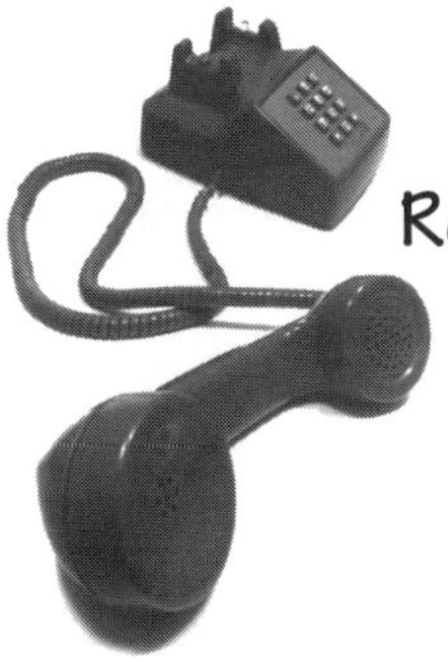

Resource Information Guide

Al-Anon/Alateen Family Group Headquarters, Inc.
1600 Corporate Landing Parkway
Virginia Beacn, VA 23454
(757) 563-1600

Alcohol Research Information Service
1106 E. Oakland
Lansing, MI 48906
(517) 485-9900

Alcoholics Anonymous World Services
P.O. Box 459, Grand Central Station
New York, NY 10163
(212) 870-3400

American Council on Alcoholism
2522 Saint Paul Street
Baltimore, MD 21218
(410) 889-0100

American Council for Drug Education (ACDE)
136 East 64th Street
New York, NY 10021
(800) 488-3784

American Medical Association (AMA)
Department of Mental Health,
Division of Substance Abuse
515 North State Street
Chicago, IL 60610
(312) 464-5000

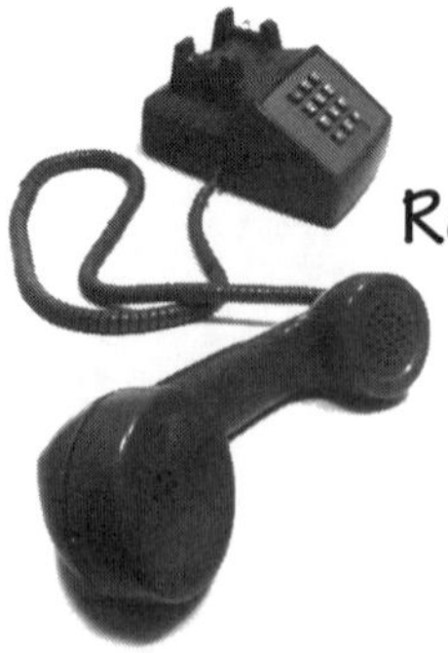

Resource Information Guide

Center for Substance Abuse Prevention (CSAP)
SAMSHA
Rockwall 2 Building, Room 9D10
5600 Fishers Lane
Rockville, MD 20857
(301) 443-0365

Center for Substance Abuse Treatment (CSAT)
SAMSHA
Rockwall 2 Building, Room 618
5600 Fishers Lane
Rockville, MD 20857
(301) 443-5700

Children of Alcoholics Foundation, Inc.
555 Madison Avenue, 20th Floor
New York, NY 10022
(212) 754-0656

Cocaine Anonymous World Services, Inc.
3740 Overland, Suite C
Los Angeles, CA 90034
(800) 347-8998

National Alcohol Hot Line
343 West Foothill Blvd.
Monrovia, CA 91016
(800) Alcohol

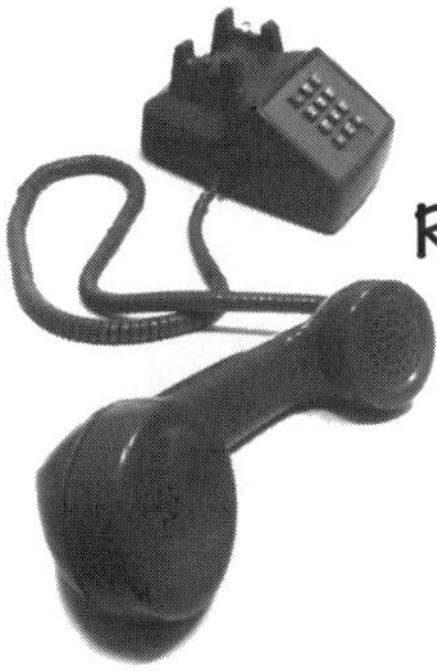

Resource Information Guide

National Council on Alcoholism
12 West 21st Street
New York, NY 10010
(212) 206-6770

National Institute On Alcohol Abuse and Alcoholism (NIAAA)
6000 Executibe Blvd., Suite 400
Bethesda, MD 20892-7003
(301) 443-3885

National Institute on Drug Abuse (NIDA)
Parklawn Building, 5600 Fisher Lane, Suite 1005
Rockville, MD 20857
(301) 443-6480

U.S. Department of Human Services
200 Independence Avenue, S.W.
Washington, D.C. 20201
(202) 619-0257

For additional assistance, check the local telephone directory under "alcoholism" or contact the local department of public health. Contact numbers are subject to change.

Responsibility: *Being accountable for one's actions and behavior without casting blame or looking for excuses.*

Career drinkers are armed with apologies, regrets, alibis, and explanations for what makes them drink. When drinkers take responsibility for their actions, they create a chance for sobriety and a new start in life.

> People are always blaming
> their circumstances for what they are.
> I don't believe in circumstances.
> The people who get on in this world
> are the people who get up and look
> for the circumstances they want
> and if they can't find them, make them.
>
> — *George Bernard Shaw*

How many times have you heard someone say, "I need a drink," or "I can't change the way I am." The "I can't" mind-set is a convenient way to shrug off responsibility. When people say, "I can't," it immediately excuses them from having to make any effort to change.

Once convinced that they can't, it becomes even more difficult to change their habits. Life can be tough enough just working on things that have a good chance of succeeding. When people entertain the notion that something is unachievable or impossible, they unnecessarily encumber themselves with negative thoughts. Removing the letter "t" from can't, moves them to a position of power.

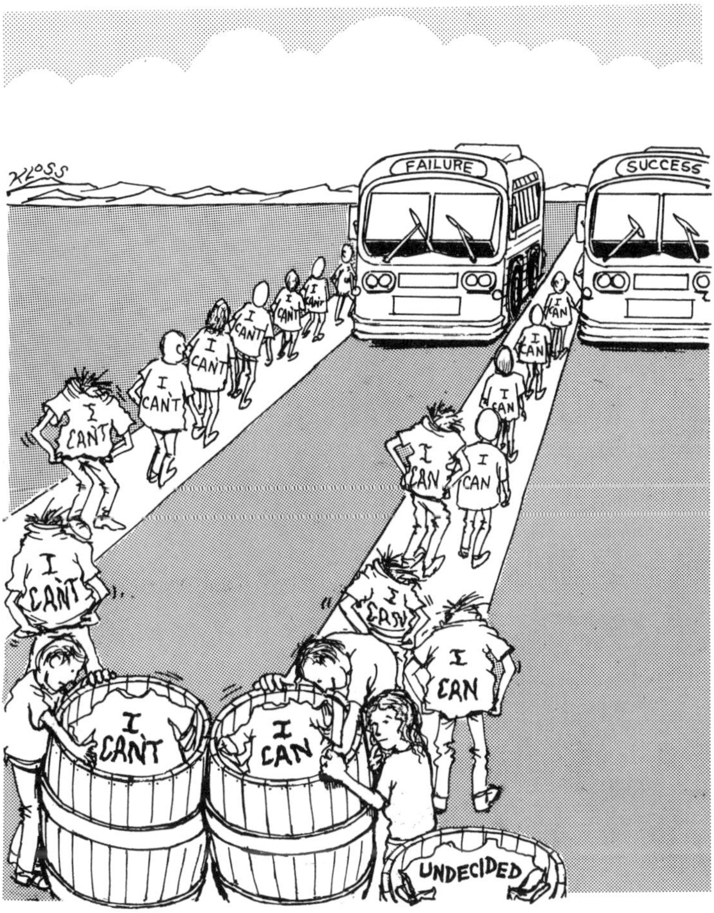

The journey begins here.

Role modeling: *Influencing the behavior of people by setting examples.* The most basic research bears out that people "do as they see," not "as they are told."

> Drunkards beget drunkards.
>
> — *Plutarch*

Parents who drink alcohol are ineffective role models if they are trying to convey the hazards of drinking to their children. It is by setting examples, not by dictating examples, that we make an impact and inspire others to be their best.

> Setting an example is not the main means of influencing another, it is the only means.
>
> — *Albert Einstein*

DID YOU KNOW?

> Peer influence may be one of the strongest predictors of alcohol use among young people.[31]

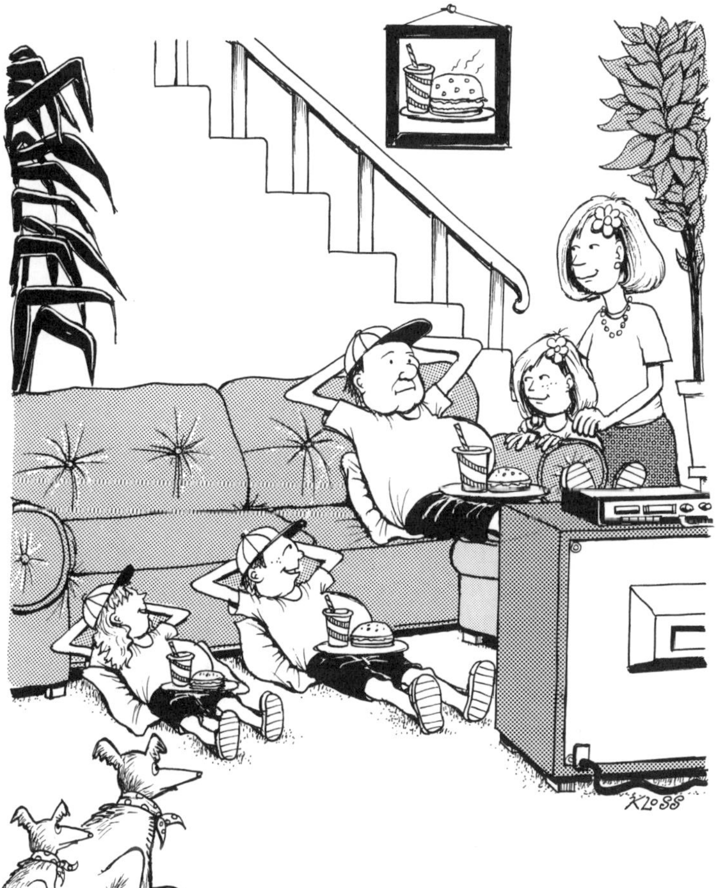

Sometimes –
Role modeling is unconscious!

Rosacea: *A condition characterized by the flushing tone and inflammation of the nose and surrounding areas.* Although the exact cause of the condition is unknown, it is often precipitated and aggravated by alcohol. In more advanced stages, a bulbous red nose develops. W.C. Fields is a classic example of a person afflicted with rosacea.

Rubbing alcohol: *A poisonous alcohol, known as isopropyl alcohol, intended for external use only.* Under no circumstances should rubbing alcohol be orally consumed.

Screening test: *A relatively easy way for determining the likelihood of a person developing a drinking problem.*

Experts recognize the CAGE screening test as one of the most effortless and practical devices used today. Developed in 1970 by Ewing and Rouse, the CAGE test quickly screens individuals for potential drinking problems. It consists of four simple questions:

CAGE Quick Screening Test

- ☐ Have you ever felt you should **C**ut down on your drinking?
- ☐ Have people **A**nnoyed you by criticizing your drinking?
- ☐ Have you ever felt bad or **G**uilty about your drinking?
- ☐ Have you ever had an **E**ye-opener first thing in the morning to steady nerves or get rid of a hangover?

If people answer "yes" to just one of the four questions above, chances are they are candidates for alcoholism. If they answered "yes" to all four questions, there is little doubt that they are alcohol dependent.

Two or three affirmative responses should evoke concern and raise suspicion. Again, keep in mind that the CAGE test is a screening process and not a diagnostic tool for devising a treatment program.

Another efficient screening tool for alcoholism is the Michigan Alcoholism Screening Test:

Michigan Alcoholism Screening Test

- ☐ Do you think you are a normal drinker? (No, 2 points)
- ☐ Have you ever awakened the morning after some drinking the night before and found that you could not remember a part of the evening? (Yes, 2 points)
- ☐ Does your wife, husband, parents, or relative ever worry or complain about your drinking? (Yes, 1 point)
- ☐ Can you stop drinking without a struggle after one or two drinks? (No, 2 points)
- ☐ Do you ever feel guilty about your drinking? (Yes, 1 point)
- ☐ Do friends or relatives think you are a normal drinker? (No, 2 points)
- ☐ Are you always able to stop drinking when you want to? (No, 2 points)
- ☐ Have you ever attended a meeting of Alcoholics Anonymous? (Yes, 5 points)
- ☐ Have you gotten into physical fights when drinking? (Yes, 1 point)
- ☐ Has drinking ever created problems between you and your wife, husband, a parent or relative? (Yes, 2 points)
- ☐ Has your wife, husband, or relative ever gone to anyone for help about your drinking? (Yes, 2 points)
- ☐ Have you ever lost any friends because of drinking? (Yes, 2 points)
- ☐ Have you ever gotten into trouble at work because of drinking? (Yes, 2 points)
- ☐ Have you ever lost a job because of drinking? (Yes, 2 points)

Continued

- [ ] Have you ever neglected your obligations, your family, or your work for two or more days in a row because you were drinking? (Yes, 2 points)
- [ ] Do you ever drink before noon? (Yes, 1 point)
- [ ] Have you ever been told that you have liver trouble? Cirrhosis? (Yes, 2 points)
- [ ] Have you ever had delirium tremens (DTs), severe shaking, heard voices or seen things that weren't there after heavy drinking? (Yes, 2 points)
- [ ] Have you ever gone to anyone for help about your drinking? (Yes, 5 points)
- [ ] Have you ever been in a hospital because of drinking? (Yes, 5 points)
- [ ] Have you ever been a patient in a psychiatric hospital or in a psychiatric ward of a general hospital where drinking was part of the problem? (Yes, 2 points)
- [ ] Have you ever been seen at a psychiatric or mental health clinic, or gone to a doctor, social worker, or clergyman for help with an emotional problem in which drinking had played a part? (Yes, 2 points)
- [ ] Have you ever been arrested, even for a few hours, because of drunk behavior? (Yes, 2 points)
- [ ] Have you ever been arrested for drunk driving or driving after drinking? (Yes, 2 points)

Original Scoring System (Screening only)

0-3 points (Nonalcoholic response)
4 points (Suggestive)
5 or more points (Alcoholic)

Adapted and reprinted with permission from the American Psychiatric Association. American Journal of Psychiatry 127: 1653-1658, 1971. Copyright 1971, the American Psychiatric Association.

Self-esteem: *A person's impression or opinion regarding self-worth.*

> What lies behind us
> and what lies before us
> are small matters compared
> to what lies within us.
>
> — *Ralph Waldo Emerson*

Some people have so little self-esteem that they fail to take care of themselves. Abusing alcohol, smoking, and eating unhealthy foods are all known to increase the risk of physical illness and diseases. These examples demonstrate how people treat themselves when they have a low perceived personal value. Take a close look at the next question.

Why would anyone buy an expensive car and then replace the motor oil with dirty motor oil? Although this seems unthinkable, many people take meticulous care of their possessions, yet neglect to take care of their most prized possessions – their inner self and their body.

It is astounding how many people have time to do subtle destructive things throughout the day, yet simply do not set aside even a fraction of their day to treat themselves well. A good example is a "stressed out" person who will not dedicate a meager two percent of a 24-hour day to relieve stress through some form of physical activity.

If we spend just two percent of the day caring for our bodies, think about the excellent condition we would be in! Incidentally, three 20-minute aerobic workouts a week represent about 1/2 of a percent of the time available in a week. When we explore intellectual ideas and open ourselves to emotional growth, we build greater respect and confidence. Dedication produces amazing results.

MYTH

Alcohol lifts spirits and boosts self-confidence.

REALITY

In light to moderate amounts, alcohol can ease inhibitions, relax the body and mind, and cause a euphoric mood for a short period of time. The opposite is true as well. In some situations, the worst behavior in someone's personality can surface.

As alcohol fades from the body, heightened feelings of euphoria and false security are usually replaced with guilt, mood swings, and low self-esteem. Excessive drinking assures deterioration of temperament, self-respect, and quality of life.

A few words about self-image

A favorable self-image is one of the most treasured and coveted attributes a person can possess. Feelings of strength, confidence, courage, and peace flourish for those who *choose* to develop their self-image.

Self-esteem is not permanently etched in stone. It is reshaped and molded with each new experience. Every day, conscious and unconscious signals are sent to the brain to evaluate self-worth. In that process, we either choose to foster positive feelings or hang on to negative feelings.

Destructive childhood experiences, abandonment, criticism, ridicule, scolding, and lack of security or love are just a few examples of what can cause feelings of low self-esteem at any age. Offering unconditional love, acceptance, patience, and encouragement can help a child or an adult grow into a self-assured individual.

Tips for Developing Self-esteem

- Encourage a person to make positive statements: "I can do it." "I can't" is no longer a part of one's vocabulary.
- Visualize things that bring joy and happiness.
- Take action on things that are important. Don't wait for things to happen.
- Take a fun, enlightening class.
- Improve nutritional habits.
- Include some fun physical activities.
- Develop one's knowledge base.
- Concentrate on one's strengths, not on perceived limitations.
- Dress for success. Buy new clothes.
- Reduce stress.

Self-fulfilling prophecy: *A prediction about oneself that becomes reality by subscribing to certain beliefs.*

> What you see as being possible,
> what you believe as being likely,
> and what you value as being sacred,
> will be who you become.
>
> — *Raymond V. Haring*

A self-fulfilling prophecy works like this: a belief about something causes a person to act accordingly. For instance, a person believes they cannot do something. Therefore, they do not try. Without trying, nothing happens. When *nothing* happens, they have proof that their self-fulfilling prophecy was accurate.

Have you ever acquired something you just knew you were going to get, whether you wanted it or not? What about those times you believed you could not do something, so you did not try? When nothing happened, you reaffirmed your self-fulfilling prophecy.

Perhaps you know someone who suffers from someone's drinking, but cannot leave. Somewhere a belief was established that reads like this: "I'm miserable and no longer have the energy to leave or change things." Believing they do not have any strength causes them to give up and accept things the way they have always been. Enduring the pain makes them even more unhappy and exhausted. They were right, they didn't have the ability or strength to change.

Coupled with defeat, their actions support their prediction. Their self-fulfilling prophecy unfolded and became reality.

A self-fulfilling prophecy does not have to be negative; it can be constructive if used in a positive way. All of us have made predictions based on past experiences and beliefs. Learn to make self-fulfilling prophecies that are health-supporting rather than limiting or self-defeating.

> Our duty as men is to proceed
> as if limits to our ability did not exist.
>
> — *Teilhard de Chardin*

Take a close look at the following table. The attitude behind each self-fulfilling prophecy reflects the difference between a winning and losing attitude:

Samples of Self-Fulfilling Prophecies

SAY YES	I prefer not to drink.
NEVER	I can't control my drinking.
SAY YES	I will meet nice people.
NEVER	I drink because I hate being alone.
SAY YES	I will enjoy my life without drinking
NEVER	I can't relax without a drink.
SAY YES	Drinking is an insignificant part of my life.
NEVER	Drinking is a huge part of my life.
SAY YES	I will succeed.
NEVER	I'm never going to make it.
SAY YES	I will do things that make me relaxed.
NEVER	I'm always stressed without a drink.
SAY YES	Life is wonderful.
NEVER	Life is tough and then you die.
SAY YES	I will be in the best shape of my life.
NEVER	I'll always be out of shape.
SAY YES	Change is easier.
NEVER	It will take me forever to change.

People should be careful what they tell themselves. People who tell themselves they can't stop drinking find it almost unbearable to quit. Throughout history, people have shaped their destiny by endorsing their self-fulfilling prophecy.

Sexual performance: *A display of sexual behavior usually communicated and more easily discussed and evaluated by consenting parties in a bedroom.*

MYTH

Alcohol stimulates sexuality.

REALITY

> Wine prepares the heart for love,
> unless you take too much.
>
> —*Ovid*

For many men and women, small amounts of alcohol can relax inhibitions, bolster confidence, and arouse sexual interest. Larger amounts of alcohol, however, encumber sexual performance. With time, a male's sexuality and masculinity can be destroyed.

DID YOU KNOW?

Heavy alcohol use among men can lead to impotence.[32]

Men who think alcohol makes them more masculine or "macho," need to think twice before drinking. Changes in hormone metabolism, caused by diminished liver function, can lead to unattractive feminine features in men. Elevated estrogen levels and decreased testosterone production cause breast enlargement and testicle shrinkage. In addition, male alcoholics show impotence, loss of libido, and decreased sperm count.

Alcohol induced hormone alterations in women are not as well understood. The direct toxic effect of alcohol on the ovaries may explain menstrual and fertility changes in women who abuse alcohol. Menstrual irregularities and ammenorrhea are additional consequences of chronic drinking.

DID YOU KNOW?

Early menopause is associated with drinking in alcoholic women.[33]

DID YOU KNOW?

Chronic alcohol abuse is associated with menstrual cycle disturbances.[34]

Shot glass: *A small glass, or jigger, used to measure approximately 1.5 ounces of liquor.*

Signs of drug abuse: *Physical, mental, and emotional indicators of potential drug abuse.*

Common Warning Signs of Drug Abuse

- Depression, moodiness, irritability or apathy
- Forgetfulness or disorientation
- Loss of appetite
- Sudden weight loss
- Sleep disorders
- Neglect of personal appearance
- Hypersensitivity
- Uncooperative behavior
- Deterioration in work performance
- Reclusive, aggressive or suicidal behavior

No attempt is made here to diagnose an individual's use or abuse of drugs. The more clues or indications, however, that one notices about a person, the more likely there is a problem with drugs.

Skin: *The outermost protective layer of body tissue.* It is considered to be the body's largest organ. Skin insulates and shields body organs from the potentially hostile environment we live in. Generally, skin cells are replaced as they are destroyed. They do, however, have their own "repair and replacement" limits from everyday wear, tear, and abuse.

Just what does our skin tell us about our health? For serious drinkers, health can be skin deep. If drinking can affect the skin's appearance, imagine the impact on the tissues beneath the skin.

Alcohol and sunlight can cause blood vessels to dilate. This can give a person a rosy, flushed look wrongly associated with "glowing" health. In truth, extra blood and nutrients are brought to the skin to repair damage.

Alcohol dilates blood vessels because it is a drug with "vasodilatation," or blood vessel widening properties. People may temporarily *look* healthier from a shot of whisky on a cold night, but the alcohol has done nothing to support their health. For the light drinker, there appears to be no major skin conditions or diseases associated with small amounts of alcohol. Chronic alcohol use is a different story. Many skin disorders can result from liver damage and poor diets caused by excessive drinking: color changes, inflammation, thinning, itching, bruising, blistering or premature aging.

Sleep: *A natural state of lowered or suspended consciousness.* Approximately one-third of our lives are gobbled up in sleep.

Normal sleep consists of various stages or cycles. Typically, a person begins the light stage of sleep by slipping into a "dozing off" phase. The next two phases are medium sleep and deep sleep, sometimes referred to as body-recovery sleep.

Dream sleep, or rapid eye movement sleep (REM), is actually a lighter level of sleep when the eyes move rapidly while dreaming. Adequate REM sleep is necessary for normal health and psychological recovery from everyday living.

MYTH

An evening drink or "nightcap" will help people get a good night's sleep.

REALITY

It is a fallacy to believe that having a few drinks, or a "nightcap," before bed will assure a good night's sleep. Although sufficient alcohol will "knock" a person out, the overall rest and recovery is inferior and fragmented.

Both deep and REM sleep are ruined with heavy episodes of drinking resulting in little normal recovery sleep. Even after eight hours in bed, a person can wake up the next morning wondering why they do not feel rested.

Sobering up: *The process of eliminating or "mopping up" alcohol in a person's system.*

MYTH

Fresh air, cold showers, and caffeine
aid the sobering process.

REALITY

It is wishful thinking that caffeinated products, fresh air, cold water, or walks around the block help sober up a person. Drinking coffee and taking a cold shower will only make a person cold, wet and concerned with emptying the bladder. As diuretics, caffeine and alcohol increase water loss in the urine. There is no home remedy for speeding the sobering process. Time is a certain cure; it is what the body needs most to destroy alcohol.

DID YOU KNOW?

Bubbles in carbonated alcoholic drinks speed up the absorption of alcohol into the blood. This explains why champagne goes to the head faster.

Sobriety: *Total abstinence from alcohol by an alcoholic.*

Maintaining sobriety is a challenge, regardless of the alcoholic's personal history. For some people, abstaining from alcohol is more than a struggle, it is literally a battle with no end. Other people, for unclear reasons, can more easily break free from the clutches of alcohol.

To minimize the risk of a relapse, it is important to

identify the high-risk factors that provoke unpleasant emotional states: situations that elicit anxiety, anger, boredom, conflict, distress, frustration or tension. They should be acknowledged and dealt with immediately. (Refer to section on *stress* for insights into dealing with stress.)

Social drinker: *A person who drinks lightly to moderately at "social" gatherings or events.* Although this term refers to a socially accepted level of drinking, it is actually too vague a term to be of much value. For some people, social drinking means just about any level of drinking when they are out celebrating or partying with friends. (Refer to section on *classification of drinking*.)

Someday: *A day sometime in the future that for certain procrastinators becomes the "eighth" day of a week or the best time to get things done.* This particular *day* could be tomorrow or sometime much later. In any event, *someday* occupies a very special time for people who avoid doing things that they believe they won't or can't do now.

Sunday, Monday, Tuesday, Wednesday,
Thursday, Friday, Saturday, **Someday...**

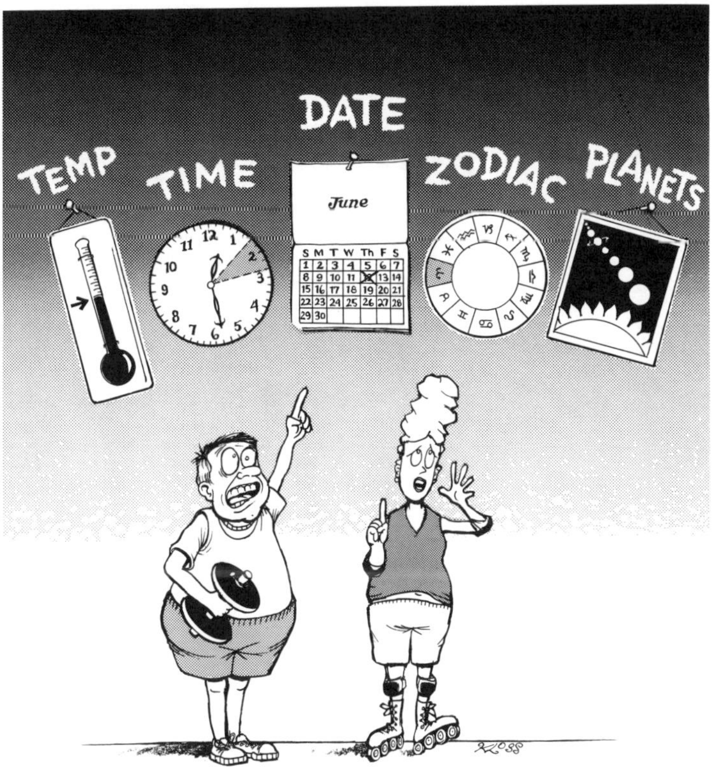

Look Honey! No more waiting – SOMEDAY has arrived with all its fury!

Sparkling wine: *Carbonated wine containing approximately 12 percent alcohol.*

Spirits: *Alcoholic beverages.*

Alcohol and Energy Content of Common Alcoholic Drinks

Beverage	Amount (Ounces)	Alcohol (Grams)	Energy (Calories)
Beer			
Regular	12	13	150
Light	12	11	90
Low alcohol	12	6.5	70
Nonalcoholic	12	1	60
Ale, malt liquor	12	15	150
Wine			
Dry wine	4	11	80
Port	4	14	190
Red	4	12	85
Sherry	4	18	150
Sweet	4	12	103
Sparkling cooler	12	12	215
Gin, rum, vodka, whiskey (94 proof)	1.5	17	115

Sports: *Games that involve physical activities.* For many people, health and physical fitness clubs have replaced smoky barrooms and nightclubs as a place to unwind. The exhilarating feeling of being healthy wins hands down over facing a nasty hangover.

For the serious sports-minded individual, alcohol use before, during, or after physical activity impairs performance. Potential problems can result from drinking alcohol: slowed reaction time, limited coordination, depressed mental alertness, and energy utilization.

Athletes and sports enthusiasts who drink alcohol before or during a sporting event are at risk for significant fluid loss. Dehydration of body tissue occurs because alcohol acts as a diuretic. It inhibits a hormone called antidiuretic hormone (ADH), necessary for instructing the kidneys to limit water excretion. Sports physicians recommend that athletes avoid alcohol, especially within 24 hours of an athletic event.

The body is made up of more than 600 different muscles. On any given day, the body makes new muscle tissue to replace "old" broken down tissues. We need to eat proteins daily so that raw building materials (amino acids) are available for rebuilding muscles. When more body proteins are being degraded than rebuilt, body muscles lose mass and strength and begin to atrophy.

Alcohol consumption increases protein degradation. Individuals with a history of heavy drinking can experience muscle damage resulting in a condition called *alcoholic myopathy* (degenerative muscle condition). It is characterized by debilitating muscle fatigue.

Tips for Building Strength, Flexibility and Endurance

Muscular strength refers to the maximum force that can be produced by an individual muscle or group of muscles. Although three general types of muscles exist: cardiac (which pumps blood), smooth (which changes the volume of stomach, uterus, etc.) and skeletal (which changes the angle of bones), most of us are usually concerned with cardiac and skeletal muscles.

Pay close attention to the following tips to increase your strength to move, lift, hold, push or pull objects heavier than you are used to moving:

- Always warm up before any workout.
- Stretch before all workouts.
- Breathe continuously – never hold your breath.
- Never train to the point of causing pain.
- Always use proper technique and equipment.
- Exercise all muscle groups.
- Use a full range of motion.
- Get adequate rest – it is just as important as activity.
- Curtail activities when you are ill.
- Seek information from professional and/or health and fitness books on the market.

Flexibility is one aspect of physical fitness that is often neglected. Flexibility is the ability to move a joint through a full nonrestricted range of motion without incurring discomfort, pain or injury. Many activities require a certain amount of flexibility. Stretching exercises are specifically designed to improve flexibility, increase the range of motion and reduce the risk of injury. Pay attention to the following tips to increase your level of flexibility:

- Slowly stretch to the point of tightness, never to the point of pain.
- Never bounce back and forth to get a stretch.
- Use caution when stretching neck and lower back muscles, as well as muscles near painful joints.
- Stretch a minimum of several times a week.
- Learn proper techniques from illustrated books.
- Whenever in doubt, ask a professional.

Muscular endurance is the ability of a muscle, or group of muscles, to contract over and over again for an extended period of time or until the muscle(s) fatigues. Most people are concerned with their cardiorespiratory (heart and lungs) endurance.

Cardiorespiratory (heart and lung) endurance, sometimes called cardiovascular endurance, is the ability of a person to persist in a physical activity for an extended length of time. Running, swimming, climbing or rowing for extended periods could certainly impose a demand on your cardiovascular, respiratory, and skeletal muscle systems. Compared to all the elements of fitness, nothing is more important than your cardiorespiratory endurance.

Our heart and lungs are two very important organs continuously delivering oxygen and nourishment to hundreds of muscles and vital organs. The benefits to good cardiorespiratory condition are phenomenal:

- Lose weight
- Improve attitude
- Reduce stress
- Improve self-esteem
- Improve general health
- Improve physical appearance
- Reduce risk of heart disease
- Develop more strength
- Feel better and more energetic
- Sleep better at night
- Become more flexible
- Increase cardiac endurance
- Enjoy more activities

Use the following table as a guide to find your training heart rate for aerobic activities:

Calculating Your Training Heart Rate for General Aerobic Activities

Step 1

220 - Age = Estimated Maximum Heart Rate (EMHR)

Step 2

(EMHR) x (%Intensity Factor) = Estimated Training Heart Rate

Note: Generally the % Intensity Factor ranges from 0.6 (Beginners) to 0.8 (Advanced). Before starting any exercise or physical fitness program it is a good idea to first see your physician.

	Beginner	Intermediate	Advanced
Duration	20 min.	30-45 min	45-60+ min.
Frequency	3x/wk.	4-5x/wk.	5-6x/wk.
Intensity	60%	70%	75-80%

Stimulants: *Chemical agents or drugs that temporarily cause mental or physical arousal.* Amphetamines (dexedrine, methamphetamine, "speed," "crank," "ice"), cocaine ("coke," "crack"), and methylphenidate (ritalin) are examples of commonly abused stimulants. Tea, coffee, and colas are commonly used stimulants because of the caffeine they contain.

MYTH

Alcohol acts as a mild stimulant
for social drinkers.

REALITY

Although alcohol is notorious for removing inhibitions, it does not stimulate brain activity. *Feeling* more socially at ease after a drink is not the same as actually *being* more alert. Ultimately, alcohol consumption at any level acts as a brain depressant.

Stress: *Feelings of anxiety, pressure, burden, and frustration as a by-product of life's daily demands.* Stress is the *response* in one's emotional, mental or physical state caused by some type of challenge. The level of stress depends on a person's perception of what has happened (or could happen) in a given circumstance.

More specifically, stress is not an *event* that happens, it is a physical, mental or emotional reaction.

There are two general categories of stress: good stress and bad stress. Bad stress, or *distress,* relates to either the actual or perceived negative event. Good stress, or *eustress,* results from a positive event.

Regardless of the situation, any event, whether viewed as positive or negative, can create stress. Losing a home or a person we love would obviously cause distress. What about the loss of a job? This could prove a curse or a blessing; it depends on our interpretation. In other words, we can view the lack of having a job as a loss or the opportunity to open new doors.

> If you are distressed by anything external,
> the pain is not due to the thing itself,
> but to your own estimate of it;
> and this you have the power
> to revoke at any moment.
>
> — *Marcus Aurelius*

Potential Sources of Stress

Physical

- Inactivity
- Injury
- Poor diet
- Insufficient sleep
- Infections
- Overweight
- Poor body image
- Drug use (abuse)
- Victimization
- Smoking
- Disease
- Disability
- Illness
- Aging

Emotional

- Change
- Disappointments
- Unresolved anger
- Unfulfilled needs
- Lack or loss of love

Social

- Being rejected, teased,
- scorned, taunted,
- ignored,
- ridiculed, deprived,
- isolated

Intellectual

- Inadequate planning
- Challenges
- Procrastination
- Inadequate education/skills
- Mental exhaustion
- Uncertainty/limbo
- Loss

Environmental

- Noise
- Population
- Pollution
- Poverty
- Climate
- Crime
- Housing
- Traffic

Spiritual

- Lack of purpose
- Moral conflicts
- Unethical behavior
- Weak beliefs (opinions)
- Lack of faith or trust
- No religion/philosophy
- Questionable values
- Out of touch with nature
- Directionless

Identifying Events that Lead to Stress

- Too much or too little work (sporadic vs. routine schedule)
- Not enough time to get things done vs. "rush and wait"
- Boring/uninteresting or unchallenging work responsibilities
- Unhealthy environment at work or home
- Personality differences (clashes) with friends or relatives
- Leisure time/vacations (planning/traveling/returning)
- Illness/disability (long vs. short-term)
- Confused/uncertain direction in life (blocked/restricted)
- Poor diet/nutritional habits (food intake/diet history)
- Death of spouse/friend/relative
- Doing things you don't want to do
- Forgetfulness
- Marriage (planning/adjustment to)
- Pregnancy (pregnant/fear of pregnancy)
- Starting/ending something (project/relationship/business)
- Fired/threat of layoff (acute or chronic anxiety or worrying)
- Social activities/responsibilities
- Career change (occupation/profession)
- Changing job (within company/to another company)

This questionnaire is not intended to be scored.
Its purpose is to help identify events that may be causing stress.

Identifying Events that Lead to Stress

- Financial problems (debts/investments/planning)
- Family/relationship problems
- Commuting/traffic problems (congestion vs. distance)
- Meeting deadlines (short vs. long-term)
- Difficulty making decisions
- Moving (changing residence)
- Divorce/separation (or fear of)
- Over/underweight/body image disorder
- Interrupted/insufficient sleep
- Personal injury (physical/emotional)
- Adjustment to retirement
- Clutter
- Procrastination
- Lack of control
- Sexual difficulties
- Poor physical fitness & health
- Additional responsibilities at work/home
- Crowded conditions (home/work/highways/desk)
- Insufficient help/lack of support/criticism of work
- Expectation of success (from yourself or from others)

This questionnaire is not intended to be scored.
Its purpose is to help identify events that may be causing stress.

Recognizing Stress Symptoms

ACTIONS/BEHAVIOR

- Excessive drinking
- Poor dietary habits
- Drug use (abuse)
- Negative/pessimistic
- Forgetful
- Change in sleep patterns
- Excessive smoking
- Rush and wait behavior
- Reckless activities
- Quick rapid speech

PHYSIOLOGICAL SYMPTOMS

- Teeth grinding
- Fatigue/easy exhaustion
- Tight chest/muscles
- Skin rashes
- Pounding/racing heart
- Constipation/diarrhea
- Cold/sweaty hands
- Excessive sweating
- Elevated blood pressure
- Shortness of breath
- Appetite change
- Upset stomach
- Eyestrain
- Headaches

EMOTIONS/FEELINGS

- Irritable
- Tense
- Intolerant
- Agitated
- Resentful
- Apathetic
- Anguish
- Low self-esteem
- Urgency
- Restless
- On-edge
- Strained
- Impatient
- Angry
- Anxious
- Lonely
- Nervous
- Easily annoyed
- Worried
- Distressed
- Emotionless

What Can Be Done About Stress?
A Quick Glance at Some Options

- Tolerate it.
Live with it.
Endure it.

A bad idea –
think of something else!

- Develop friendships and support groups.

Very helpful –
even if you are not stressed!

- Hope that it will go away.
Do nothing.

Not a great plan –
having hope is great, but
taking action relieves stress!

- Learn to relax.

Fantastic idea –
have some fun, bring out
the kid in you!

- Put stressful events into perspective – is the stress real or imagined?
Change the way you think about stressful events.

A wonderful idea –
most stress and fears we
experience are imagined.

- Seek professional guidance.

A possibility –
sometimes not an option.

- Learn to verbalize and deal with your feelings.

A comforting approach –
a stress buster!

- Learn how to manage and cope with stressful events.

A great strategy –
sometimes the only option we have.

- Simply withdraw.
Avoid stressful circumstances, surroundings, and events at all costs.

Not the best option –
naps, baths, vacations and "rest"
are extremely helpful!

Activities to Reduce Stress

Aerobics	Garden	Watch people
Eat/dine	Read	Travel
Listen to music	Write	Dance
Watch television	Sail	Massage
Run	Swim	Tennis
Walk	Cook/bake	Bowl
Weight train	Baseball	Board games
Daydream	Movies	Carpentry
Public Speaking	Paint	Publish articles
Shop	Rest	Bird watch
Golf	Jump rope	Soccer
Talk with friends	Nap/sleep	Wrestle
Make handicrafts	Row	Yoga
Take baths/sauna	Basketball	Volleyball
Gymnastics	Martial arts	Stretch
Meditation	Ski	Work (of any kind)
Snowshoe	Fish	Horseback ride
Sit/rock	Knit/sew	Crossword puzzles
Help others	Think	Other . . .

Synergistic effect: *An interaction between drugs wherein one drug enhances the effect of the other.* (Refer to section on *drug and alcohol interactions* for more details.)

Teetotaler: *A person who never drinks alcohol.*

Thoughts: *Images and ideas that we process and ponder.*

Never underestimate the power of a single thought. A single thought can make the difference between destroying a life or bringing about enormous success.

> A moment's insight is sometimes worth a life's experience.
>
> — *Oliver Wendell Holmes*

What are your thoughts about alcohol? What mind-set prompts people to abuse alcohol? What insights tell them to stop abusing alcohol? Answers to these questions can profoundly influence the pattern of drinking in a person's life and, ultimately, the direction of their life.

Thoughts are shaped by experiences and supported by beliefs. Today's thoughts will be reflected in tomorrow's actions. Changing thoughts can and does change lives.

This may sound too simplistic, but if we want to change, we must begin by looking closely at the quality of our thoughts. Being in charge puts us in the driver's seat to deal with any challenges that may lie ahead.

> Our achievements of today
> are but the sum total
> of our thoughts of yesterday.
> You are today where the thoughts
> of yesterday have brought you
> and will be tomorrow
> where the thoughts of today take you.
>
> — *Blaise Pascal*

Tobacco*: Plant leaves harvested from various species of nicotiana (any of several types of tobacco plants, including nicotiana tobacum). Nicotiana tobacum* is the major type of tobacco plant grown around the world. The leaves of cultivated tobacco plants have for centuries been commercially prepared for smoking and chewing.

Nicotine is the addictive chemical substance in tobacco that is primarily responsible for tobacco dependence that develops with repeated use. Inhalation of tobacco smoke is the most effective drug-delivery system for nicotine intake. Smoking one cigarette is the equivalent of intravenously injecting between one and three milligrams of nicotine.

Aside from the addictive nature of nicotine, it is one of the most toxic drugs consumed. In addition to nicotine, tobacco smoke contains more than 4,000 chemical compounds; more than 40 of which are known cancer causing agents.

New research continues to shed light on why nicotine and other powerful drugs such as alcohol, cocaine, heroin, and amphetamines are addicting. The answer to the mysterious chain of events that contributes to a chemical dependency lies in unraveling the intricate links between physiological and chemical processes occurring inside certain brain cells. One of the hottest areas in addiction research focuses on the role certain brain *messenger* chemicals or neurotransmitters play in chemical dependency. One such neurotransmitter receiving attention is dopamine.

For years, it has been known that dopamine is intricately involved in the transmission of brain signals that not only affect behavior and learning, but also produce very pleasurable feelings when released into the synapses of brain cells. Recently, however, the interrelation between elevated dopamine levels and chemical dependency is getting huge attention by scientists. Continuing research will ultimately determine the influence various drugs have on effecting dopamine levels in the brain, and dopamine's association with chemical dependency.

MYTH

Low-tar and nicotine cigarettes are less dangerous than higher-tar and nicotine cigarettes.

REALITY

To compensate for lower levels of tar and nicotine in certain cigarettes, smokers tend to inhale more deeply and smoke more often.

According to the American Cancer Society, inhaling smoke from burning tobacco is considered the largest single preventable cause of disability and death in the United States. The American Cancer Society further asserts that tobacco use contributes to nearly one in five deaths in the United States. Smoking, aside from being one of the major causes of heart disease, is also responsible for nearly 90 percent of all cases of lung cancer.

DID YOU KNOW?

Environmental or second hand smoke that comes from the lit end of a cigarette or cigar, technically referred to as "sidestream smoke," is the smoke inhaled by anyone in the vicinity of the smoker. Convincing evidence has linked environmental tobacco smoke exposure to an alarming number of health related problems in persons exposed to this smoke.

Common Health Risks Associated with Tobacco Use:

- Cardiovascular and pulmonary diseases
- Chronic obstructive lung disease
- Chronic cough and mucus secretion
- Strokes, cataracts, reduced wound healing
- Bladder, kidney, lung, cervical, stomach, intestinal, pancreatic, oral, and pharyngeal cancer

Tobacco, smokeless: *Includes chewing tobacco and snuff.* Chewing tobacco is leaf tobacco that is sucked and occasionally chewed, but generally not swallowed. Snuff is finely shredded smokeless tobacco.

MYTH

Use of smokeless tobacco is safer than inhaling tobacco smoke.

REALITY

From all reports, smokeless tobacco is as addicting and dangerous as smoking tobacco. Whether the hazardous chemicals and toxins are absorbed via the lungs by smoking or absorbed through the mouth and intestinal track after chewing the tobacco, the addictive and cancer causing agents go to work on the human body.

Effects of Smokeless Tobacco:

- Nicotine addiction
- Cancer of the mouth, lips, tongue, cheek, and throat
- Gum disease and tooth decay
- Increased heart rate and blood pressure
- Damage to membrane lining of the mouth and throat
- Blood vessel constriction
- Depressed sense of taste and smell
- Bad breath

Tolerance: *A condition created by increased drug use that alters a person's metabolism in such a way that a higher drug dose is required in order to produce a similar effect that was achieved earlier with lesser amounts.* Increased alcohol tolerance is a key indicator of abuse and dependence. It is a banner waving DANGER AHEAD.

Tolerance develops with continuous drug use. The body tissues become less sensitive to the drug, and/or the liver becomes more efficient at degrading the drug.

Chronic alcohol use can also lead to *cross-tolerance:* a tolerance that has been extended or transferred to another drug.

Toxicity: *The quality of something poisonous or harmful to the body.* Any drug, regardless of its intended use, can become toxic to the body if consumed in sufficient quantities.

Generally, because of the wide acceptance of certain drugs and alcohol, many people do not fully realize the harmful effects caused by their continued use.

MYTH

Cheap wine or liquor is more harmful
to the body than expensive liquor or beer.

REALITY

There is only one kind of alcohol produced by the fermentation of sugars. We usually refer to it as alcohol. Its technical name is ethanol or ethyl alcohol.

The cost of a bottle of liquor has nothing to do with the quality of the alcohol. All alcoholic drinks have the same compound. Differences can occur in the quality of alcoholic beverages based on their age and on the presence of additives or products formed during their processing. Regardless of the source of the alcohol, the long-term, detrimental effects of alcohol are associated with the dose, frequency, and duration of drinking.

Treatment: *Any kind of therapy that improves a person's mental, physical, or spiritual condition.*

No one needs to be absolutely certain that someone is an alcoholic or has a major problem before they take action or offer help. Early intervention will prevent a small problem from developing into one that is far less manageable.

Do these words sound familiar? "How can Jim have a drinking problem? He hasn't missed a day of work," or "Judy doesn't act like an alcoholic. She just enjoys drinking like the rest of her friends."

We are waiting too long if we are looking for the drinker to "cross the line" or do something that unequivocally indicates alcohol abuse. We need to take immediate action if we have a concern or even suspect that a drinking problem is developing. Alcohol use does not have to be out of control or devastating before help can be provided.

A first step might be a telephone call to a local mental health facility, hospital, or alcoholism treatment center. Many health care professionals are drug abuse specialists, providing the best possible advice and care to those willing to listen and accept help. It has been said, "Where there is a will, there is a way." Help is available for those who want to change their lives.

Health field professionals realize that the first step toward recovery for drinkers is their acceptance of a drinking problem. "Denial" is commonly used by many alcoholics to avoid seeking help.

A procedure called *intervention* is a useful method for persuading drinkers that they have a drinking problem and are in need of professional help. Counselors, family members and close friends meet with drinkers to explain how alcohol is destroying the quality of life for all concerned. The main objective of intervention is to convince the alcoholic to get immediate treatment.

Seek medical advice if there is doubt about the severity of alcohol dependence. Generally, *detoxification* is the beginning of a treatment program for someone with a serious alcohol problem. Detoxification is the process of eliminating all traces of alcohol from the body. Medical supervision is generally recommended in more serious cases. Although the risk varies, life-threatening withdrawal symptoms can occur when the body is abruptly deprived of a drug upon which it is dependent.

After detoxification, many alcoholics seek outpatient treatment coupled with regular attendance at Alcoholics Anonymous meetings. Outpatient treatment programs usually require the alcoholic to attend nightly group counseling sessions for several months. In many cases, patients find it useful to attend Alcoholics Anonymous meetings in addition to regular outpatient counseling.

In more advanced stages of alcoholism, the alcoholic may wish to get help from an inpatient therapy program before seeking additional therapy. Inpatient therapy usually lasts approximately four to six weeks. Regardless of initial treatment sought, it is important to understand that the alcoholic is in the early stage of recovery.

Alcoholism is never cured. It can, however, be arrested with diligent treatment and patience. Long-term therapy involves rebuilding self-esteem and learning how to cope with the myriad of emotions that may have contributed to the person's alcohol abuse. Learning to deal with loneliness, anger, stress, frustration, shame, and guilt is an important phase in reconstructing a satisfying and fulfilling life free of alcohol.

Signs that Inpatient Care is Generally Recommended

- Potential medical problems exist
- Minimal or no family and social support groups
- Risk of serious withdrawal
- Significant resistance or ambivalence toward therapy
- Recommended by health professionals
- Unsuccessful attempts to stop drinking with outpatient programs

Signs that Outpatient Care is Generally Recommended

- Medical problems or complications do not exist
- Slight risk of serious health complications from withdrawal
- Adequate social and family support
- No history of unsuccessful attempts to stop drinking
- Recognition that a drinking problem exists and therapy is needed
- Recommended by a health professional

How to Choose a Treatment Clinic

There are thousands of alcohol treatment clinics around the country. In every state there are many nonprofit and profit clinics available. Choosing the right treatment center is important. The following questions may help assist in selecting the appropriate center:

- Is the facility accredited and licensed by the state?
- What is the nature of the treatment program?
- Are follow-up treatment and support offered?
- Will the cost of treatment be covered by insurance?
- Is the facility recognized by the Joint Commission on Accreditation of Hospitals?
- Will a chapter of the National Council on Alcoholism recommend the facility?

Tunnel vision: *A point of view so restrictive that virtually one idea or thought occupies the brain for extended periods of time.* Some people dwell on things until they become obsessed, ill, or feel they need a drink to escape.

Tunnel vision has been called the "one-track" mind syndrome. When people view things with tunnel vision, they miss everything, much like walking through an art museum while looking at their feet.

The concept of victimization is an example of tunnel vision carried to an extreme. Victimized people view themselves as helpless and unable to see alternatives for living their lives fully. They seem paralyzed with false beliefs that restrict and prevent positive change.

The end of tunnel vision begins with an awareness of new possibilities. People previously held captive by fear can find new direction by broadening their beliefs. Falsely perceived, groundless thoughts are inherent in many fears.

> Some of your hurts you have cured,
> and the sharpest you still have survived,
> but what torments of grief you endured,
> from evils that never arrived.
>
> — *Ralph Waldo Emerson*

Twelve-Step Program: *Twelve basic steps outlined by Alcoholics Anonymous used as a guide for any alcohol treatment or recovery program.*

The Twelve Steps of AA

- We admitted we were powerless over alcohol — that our lives had become unmanageable.
- Came to believe that a Power greater than ourselves could restore us to sanity.
- Made a decision to turn our will and our lives over to the care of God, as we understood Him.
- Made a searching and fearless moral inventory of ourselves.
- Admitted to God, to ourselves, and to another human being the exact nature of our wrongs.
- Were entirely ready to have God remove all these defects of character.
- Humbly asked Him to remove our shortcomings.
- Made a list of all persons we harmed, and became willing to make amends to them all.
- Made direct amends to such people wherever possible, except when to do so would injure them or others.
- Continued to take personal inventory and when we were wrong, promptly admitted it.
- Sought through prayer and meditation to improve our conscious contact with God, as we understood Him, praying only for knowledge of His will for us and the power to carry that out.
- Having had a spiritual awakening as the result of these steps, we tried to carry this message to alcoholics and to practice these principles in all our affairs.

Ulcers: *An internal or external open sore characterized by cell destruction.* Gastric ulcers refer to open sores in the stomach.

Alcohol is an irritant to the lining of the stomach. It also stimulates the flow of digestive juices and hydrochloric acid. People suffering from ulcers, especially gastric ulcers, should avoid alcohol use.

DID YOU KNOW?

> The common ulcer drug cimetidine (Tagamet), actually decreases the ability of the stomach to burn alcohol. This can translate to higher levels of alcohol circulating in the blood and brain.

Values: *Principles held in high regard.* Simply put, what we value possesses a certain degree of desirability. Consequently, values determine decisions, give guidance, and provide meaning to life's pursuits.

> What you value is what you think about.
> What you think about is what you become.
>
> —*Joel Weldon*

We all have values. Some values include good health, a great job, a happy home life, spare time, close friendships, and money. While the list goes on, the important point is that the degree of desirability determines the relative importance of the value.

Often, due to time constraints or lack of resources, people are forced to prioritize their values. To seek their highest level of happiness and wellness, they must determine what they value most, and then commit to live by those values each day. When drinking does not support their values, it is time to reevaluate where alcohol fits into their life.

The following table may be useful in prioritizing values:

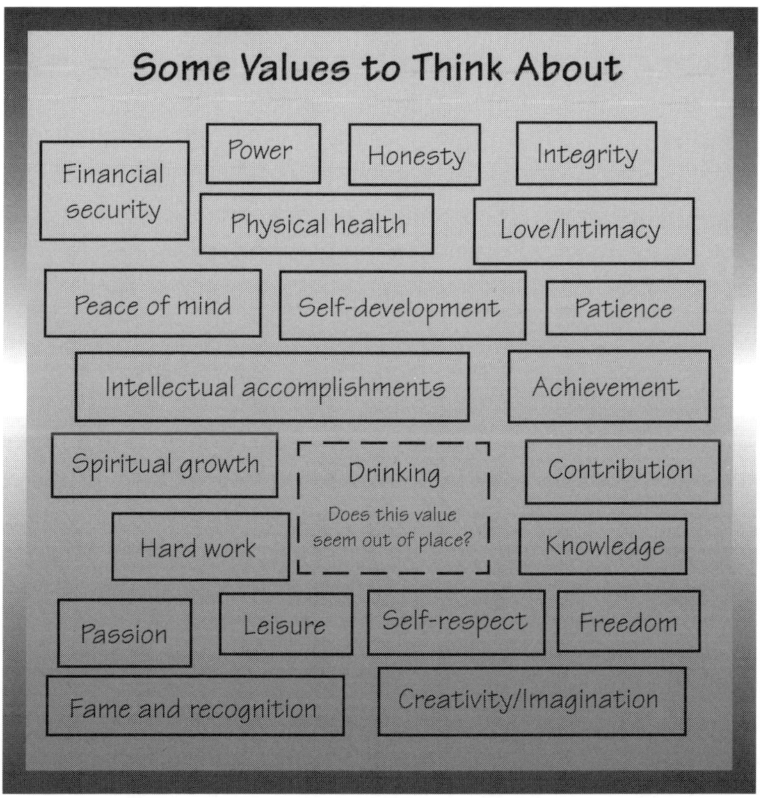

DID YOU KNOW?

A value, unsupported by rules and limits, is like a table without legs. There is nothing to stand on. Consider the person who wants a healthy heart but who still consumes unhealthy foods, or the drinker who wants to quit drinking between drinks. *Thinking* about a value is much different than *living* it.

If people are unsure about what they value, they need to look at what they are doing. What a person does *is* what they value. If drinking is a significant part of their social lives, then alcohol has value and importance to them.

Visualization: *Imagining what has happened or could happen.*

> Nothing happens unless first a dream.
>
> — *Carl Sandburg*

Visualization is nothing new. People have been doing it for years, perhaps without knowing its immeasurable influence on their lives. Thoughts, memories, daydreams, fantasies, impressions, and dreams are examples of the visualization process.

As a powerful vehicle for change, visualization helps people to reduce stress, overcome fears, improve self-esteem, achieve goals, and abstain from alcohol.

Some people see themselves as victims and hold

themselves hostage to pain and suffering. Other people see themselves as visionaries who believe nothing is impossible. As dreamers, they have the freedom to shape their own lives and quite possibly, the lives of others.

Visualization means power. Although it cannot perform miracles or force someone to stop drinking, it remains, however, one of the best ways to gain insight and find solutions to problems. Imagery is like a tour guide helping people find clear directions in their journeys.

> Imagination is more important than knowledge.
>
> — *Albert Einstein*

Visualization, however, can have two sides: one positive and the other negative. People who suffer from anxiety, worry, fear, and stress have mastered the unfavorable side of visualization. They see things that cause distress. Some alcoholics and ulcer patients are *grand masters* at visualizing things that cause anxiety and worry.

Other people who apply the positive side of visualization create life's marvels of health, happiness, and peace of mind.

Want: *A desire as weak as a wish or as strong as a commitment.*

The word *want* is often misunderstood, yet a good grasp of its meaning can change our lives. Examine the various meanings in the definitions below:

- *Wishing, hoping, dreaming or longing for something*
- *Expressing a casual interest*
- *Having a curiosity*
- *Having an earnest desire*
- *Feeling a need*
- *Being determined*
- *Having an unwavering commitment to work toward a goal*

Although all of the definitions imply an interest in something, the actual intent behind each expression may be worlds apart.

If people say they *wish* to stop drinking, that statement is not as strong as those who assert, "I will stop drinking and absolutely nothing will stand in my way."

The point is simple. If people want something, they need to make a firm commitment to see that the goal is accomplished.

Weight control: *Regulating food intake and energy expenditure to achieve and maintain a desired weight and body composition.* Weight control involves more than simply doing "extra" exercises and eating less food. The success of any diet ultimately hinges on unique circumstances.

People should consider their attitude they have about food. Are they eating or drinking because of loneliness, boredom, or depression? If they are not hungry or thirsty, this may be their first clue that there is an underlying problem.

Part of dieting is eliminating or curtailing the intake of alcoholic beverages. Weight loss and drinking alcohol do not mix well. Alcohol is a strong central nervous system or brain depressant and tends to curb enthusiasm for mental and physical activities. With each alcoholic drink consumed, interest in physical activity plummets along with drive and ambition to diet.

The following statements summarize the major points concerning dieting and weight loss:

The Seven Golden Rules for Weight Loss

Don't drink alcohol. Alcohol is extremely fattening. Its high energy and "chemical" content send instructions to the liver to make fat.

Alcohol has an entirely different look on the body than it does in a bottle or glass.

Eat a high starch-based plant diet from different foods. This adds balance and variety to assure adequate intake of important essential nutrients. A high starch-based diet is low in fat and contains little or no cholesterol. People may even get tired of eating. They will no longer be able to say, "I hardly eat and I gain weight." They will be eating all the time.

What we eat can be more important than how much we eat.

Eliminate fat from the diet wherever possible. Fatty sauces and toppings must be significantly reduced. Diets do not work if people begin eating fatty foods. Fats are extremely high in calories and love to live in "little" fat stores on the thighs, belly, waist, and chin.

What we don't eat can be as important as what we do eat.

Exercise! Start thinking about the shape and condition of the body and less about weight; the weight issue will take care of itself as we become more physically fit.

Transfer the weight from the waist, chin and buttocks to the biceps, shoulders and other body muscles for a tapered fit look.

The best way to lose fat is to exercise aerobically for at least 20 minutes several times a week. Any activity qualifies as aerobic when the heart rate has reached a certain point. (See section on sports.)

Don't lose weight too quickly. Losing weight too rapidly destroys valuable muscle tissue that acts as powerful "fat burners." Focus on losing body fat, not on losing muscle and body tone.

Muscle tissue is our best friend in losing flabby pounds. Muscle tissue thrives on burning energy – especially when we put our muscles to work. Unlike fat tissue, muscle burns tremendous amounts of energy, even when our muscles are resting. Trying to lose weight when losing muscle tissue is like trying to sail without wind in the sails – it's futile.

Fat tissue thrives on storing energy. The more fat we wear,

the more fat cells love to be fed. Fat cells have a ravenous appetite in maintaining their physique. A vicious cycle of weight gain may ensue. If we become inactive, our fat cells will work overtime to turn us into chubby balls of fat.

Avoid exotic diets. Shy away from diets made up of expensive or unusual foods that make diets difficult to follow and adhere to. Foods should also be readily available and affordable. There are no magical formulations or particular foods that will help the body burn fat faster.

Choose a diet plan for life. Who wants to lose weight only to gain it back? There are two phases to weight loss: losing the weight and keeping it from returning.

Changing diet and life-style confronts both issues. It would be wonderful to receive a diploma that keeps weight from returning. Unfortunately, no such certificate exists. Weight, health, and fitness are always subject to change.

Be patient. It takes time to gain weight, so it's going to take time to lose it. Avoid starvation or very low energy diets. Any diet will ultimately fail if it makes a person feel hungry and weak.

Permanent weight loss involves life-style changes. Big dividends are ahead for those people who modify their attitudes, habits, and beliefs about food.

Well-being: *A condition of health, happiness, and prosperity achieved through physical, mental, and spiritual growth.* Growth comes from facing challenges and overcoming them.

When people treat daily challenges as problems, they tend to surrender their well-being and sense of inner peace. Coupled with stress and anxiety, their behavior is encouraged by drinking.

Wellness: *A state of well-being developed by taking responsibility for life-style behaviors that promote well-being.*

Old Behaviors That Do Not Support Health

____

____

____

____

____

____

____

____

____

____

____

____

New Behaviors That Support Health

Wernicke-Korsakoff syndrome: *Two forms of brain disease associated with malnutrition and long-term abuse of alcohol.* Although separate conditions, both are often discussed together as one syndrome.

Amnesia is usually so severe in Korsakoff's syndrome, that confabulating (inventing stories) is used as a means of coping with the victim's inability to recall past events or to process new material.

Wernicke's syndrome results from a thiamine deficiency caused by poor diet and alcohol ingestion. Some of the major symptoms include: nystagmus (abnormal eye movements), ataxia (difficulty with muscular coordination, especially walking), disorientation, and confusion.

Wine: *An alcoholic beverage made from fermented grapes.* The two basic types of wine made from grapes are *generic* and *varietal* blends. Burgundy, Chablis, and Rhine are examples of *generic* wines made from blending a mixture of different wine grapes.

Varietal wines, such as Chardonnay and Zinfandel, are made from at least 51 percent of one type of grape.

White wines are usually made from white grapes or from skinless red grapes. Red wines are produced from crushed, unpeeled red grapes. Rose wines can be made by mixing white and red wines or by leaving the red grape skins in the fermentation process for a day or two. The "drier" wines contain less sugar.

Carbon dioxide bubbles are made during fermentation. Sparkling wines and Champagne can be made naturally by mixing a small amount of sugar to the wine during the bottling stage.

DID YOU KNOW?

The alcohol content of most wines is approximately 10 percent by volume. Fortified wines, those that have additional alcohol added, average about 20 percent alcohol by volume.

Wishing well: *A place in our minds where hope is given a chance to succeed.* Wishing and hoping for health are passive activities requiring little effort and producing even fewer results.

> A consistent man believes in destiny,
> a capricious man in chance.
>
> — *Benjamin Disraeli*

Without effort and commitment, fitness and health goals remain nothing more than daydreams. The quality and direction of our lives are dependent on simple things we do each and every day. Satisfying a goal, regardless of its nature or size, is achieved by taking one small step at a time.

> The first beginnings of things
> cannot be distinguished by the eye.
>
> — *Lucretius 99-55 B.C.*

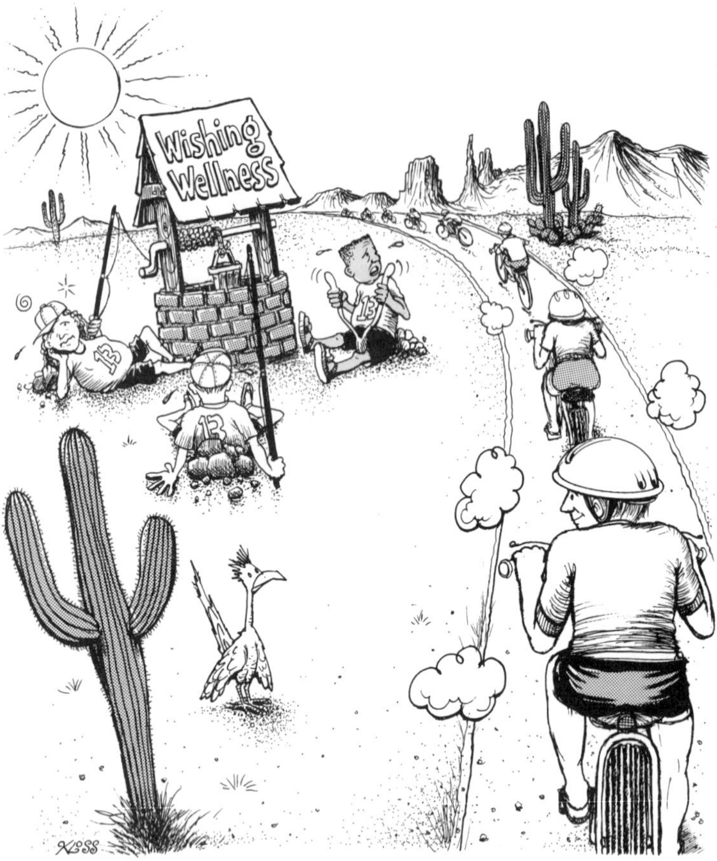

Amazing how dreams come true.

Withdrawal: *The physiological reaction of the body when deprived of a substance to which it has developed a dependence.*

Based on the history of alcohol abuse, withdrawal symptoms can be markedly different. In general, the intensity of withdrawal symptoms is dependent on dose, duration, and frequency of alcohol use. In the early phase, withdrawal symptoms usually include: headaches, irritability, anxiety, craving for alcohol, nausea, tremors, insomnia, and some degree of impaired short-term memory loss.

Symptoms may begin as early as several hours after drinking has ceased. On average, withdrawal symptoms follow a sharp decline in blood alcohol levels, which both occur within four to 12 hours after alcohol consumption has diminished or stopped.

MYTH

When alcoholics try to quit drinking,
they have "alcohol withdrawal" conditions resembling
"Rum Fits," "DTs," and grand mal seizures.

REALITY

Less than five percent of drinkers develop the horrifying symptoms manifested with the DTs and convulsive seizures.

As a general rule, the *acute* withdrawal process usually lasts several days to a week. Immediately following this stage, less severe symptoms of anxiety, insomnia, depression, irritability, loss of appetite, and other general physical symptoms may last for several weeks or months.

Candidates More Likely to Experience DTs

- Chronic drinking for 10 years or more
- Heavy drinking up to point of abstinence
- Abuse of barbiturates or other sedatives
- Previous history of DTs upon abstinence

DID YOU KNOW?

"Rum Fits," or convulsive seizures, typically begin within a few days of abstinence. Although convulsive seizures characterize an intense reaction to withdrawal, they are generally considered less serious than the DTs.

Cessation of drinking during the advanced stages of alcoholism can result in delirium tremens, or DTs, the most serious set of withdrawal symptoms known. Hallucinations, uncontrolled violent muscle contractions and trembling, nausea, severe agitation, and varying degrees of mental confusion are some of the major symptoms that usually last several days before subsiding.

The American Psychiatric Association's current *Diagnostic and Statistical Manual (DSM-IV)* describes the criteria used to diagnose alcohol withdrawal:

Diagnostic Criteria for Alcohol Withdrawal

The American Psychiatric Association's Diagnostic and Statistical Manual *DSM-IV* outlines criteria used to diagnose Alcohol Withdrawal.

Group A Response:

- [ ] Suspension or reduction in alcohol consumption after drinking has been excessive and prolonged.

Group B Response:

- [ ] Two or more of the following symptoms appearing within several hours to a few days after quitting or reducing alcohol intake after it has been excessive and prolonged.

  – anxiety
  – intensified hand tremor
  – insomnia (sleep disorder)
  – nausea or vomiting
  – grand mal seizures
  – psychomotor agitation
  – transient auditory, visual or tactile hallucinations or illusions.
  – "autonomic hyperactivity," sweating or heart beats above 100 per minute.

Group C Response:

- [ ] The symptoms in group B significantly impair or cause distress in occupational, social or other important areas of living.

Group D Response:

- [ ] The symptoms above are not a result of an existing medical condition or another mental disorder.

Note: Criteria A-D are essential features of Alcohol Withdrawal. "With Perceptual Disturbances" can be noted when hallucinations or illusions occur. The degree of alcohol withdrawal is related to the severity of symptoms.

Worry: *Exaggerated concern with impending or imaginary situations.* Worrying is a process of focusing thoughts on things that appear threatening, whether real or imagined.

> As a rule, men worry more about
> what they can't see
> than about what they can.
>
> — *Julius Caesar*

Worrying produces no results and offers no solutions. If people have a drinking problem, or know of someone who does, they might want to consider the following suggestion: spend more time finding solutions and less time worrying about problems. **Life is either too short or too long to worry.**

> Now this is not the end.
> It is not even the beginning of the end.
> But it is, perhaps,
> the end of the beginning.
>
> — *Sir Winston Churchill*

REFERENCES

1. Hill, S.Y. Vulnerability to the biochemical consequences of alcoholism and alcohol-related problems among women. In: Wilsnack, S.C., and Beckman, L.J., eds. *Alcohol Problems in Women. Antecedents, consequences, and intervention.* New York: Guilford Press, 1984. pp. 121-154.

2. Frezza, M.; DiPadova, C.; Pozzato, G.; Terpin, M.; Baraona, E.; and Lieber, C.S. High blood alcohol levels in women: The role of decreased gastric alcohol dehydrogenase activity and first-pass metabolism. *New England Journal of Medicine* 322(2): pp. 95-99, 1990.

3. NIAAAA, *Sixth Special Report to U.S. Congress on Alcohol and Health.* op.cit., p. 3, 1987.

4. *U.S. Pharmacist*, The pharmacodynamics of alcohol, Jobson Publishing Corporation, 100 Avenue of the Americas, New York, New York, February 1992.

5. Helzer, J.E.; Burman, A.; and McEvoy, L.T. Alcohol abuse and dependency. In: Robins, L.N., and Regier, D.A., eds. *Psychiatric Disorders in America: The epidemiologic catchment study.* New York: Free Press, pp. 81-115, 1991.

6. Shinn, A.F., and Shrewsbury, R.P., eds. *Evaluations of Drug Interactions.* New York: MacMillan, 1988.

7. J.G. Modell and J.M. Mountz. Drinking and flying – The problem of alcohol use by pilots. *The New England Journal of Medicine* 323 (7): pp. 455-461, 1990.

8. Cohen, E.J.; Klatsky, A.L.; and Armstrong, M.A. Alcohol use and superventricular arrhythmia. *Am J Cardiology* 62(13): pp. 971-973, 1988.

9. General Service Office of Alcoholics Anonymous, 1989 Membership Survey, preliminary results.

10. NIAAA, *Eighth Special Report to the U.S. Congress on Alcohol and Health*, op.cit., p. 165, 1993.

11. J. Leland. In: Alcohol use and abuse in ethnic minority women, eds. S. Wilsnack and L. Beckman, *Alcohol Problems in Women* (New York: The Guilford Press, 1984), p. 78.

12. Grant, B.F.; Dufour, M.C.; and Hartford, T.C. Epidemiology of liver disease. *Semin Liver Dis* 8(1): pp. 12-25, 1988.

13. Williams, G.D., and DeBakey, S.F. Changes in levels of alcohol consumption: United States, 1983 to 1988. *Br J Addict* 87(4): pp. 643-648, 1992.

14. Zador, P.L. Alcohol-related relative risk of fatal driver injuries in relation to driver and age and sex. *J Stud Alcohol* 52(4): pp. 302-310, 1991.

15. NIAAAA, *Seventh Special Report to U.S. Congress on Alcohol and Health*, op.cit., pp. 163-167, 1990.

16. National Highway Traffic Administration, *Fatal accident reporting system*, 1988, Washington, DC.

17. Leiber, C.S., *Medical and nutritional complications of alcoholism: Mechanisms in management.* New York: Plenum Publishing Corp., 1992. pp. 515-530.

18. Pequignot, G.; Tuyns, A.J.; and Berta, J.L. Ascitic cirrhosis in relation to alcohol consumption. *Int J Epidemiol* 7(2): pp. 113-120, 1978.

19. Mezey, E.; Kolman, C.J.; Diehl, A.M.; Mitchell, M.C.; and Herlong, H.F. Alcohol and dietary intake in the development of pancreatitis and liver disease in alcoholism. *Am J Clin Nutr* 48: pp. 148-151, 1988.

20. Sokol. R.J.; Ager, J.; Martier, S.; Debanne, S.; Ernhart, C.; Kuzma, J.; & Miller, S.I. Significant determinants of susceptibility to alcohol teratogenicity. *Annals of the New York Academy of Sciences* 477: pp. 87-102, 1986.

21. Harwood, H.J., and Napolitano, D.M. Economic implications of the fetal alcohol syndrome. *Alcohol Health Res World* 10(1): pp. 38-43, 1985.

22. National Institute on Alcohol Abuse and Alcoholism. In: *Eighth Special Report to the U.S. Congress on Alcohol and Health.* NIH Pub. No. 94-3699. Bethesda, MD: National Institute of Health, 1993. pp. 62-65.

23. Lands, W.E.M., and Zakhari, S. Alcohol and cardiovascualr disease. *Alcohol Health Res World* 14(4): pp. 304-312, 1990.

24. Witteman, J.C.M.; Willett, W.C.; Stampfer, M.J.; Colditz, G.A.; Kok, F.J.; Sacks, F.M.; Speizer, F.E.; Rosner, B.; and Hennekens, C.H. Relation of moderate alcohol consumption and risk of systemic hypertension in women. *Am J Cardiology* 65(9): pp. 633-637, 1990.

25. Witteman, J.C.M.; Willett, W.C.; Stampfer, M.J.; Colditz, G.A.; Kok, F.J.; Sacks, F.M.; Speizer, F.E.; Rosner, B.; and Hennekens, C.H. Relation of Moderate Alcohol Consumption and Risk of Systemic Hypertension in Women. *Am J Cardiology* 65(9): pp. 633-637, 1990.

26. Gorelick, P.B. The status of alcohol as a risk factor for stroke. *Stroke* 20(12): pp. 1607-1610, 1989.

27. *U.S. Pharmacist*, The pharmacodynamics of alcohol, Jobson Publishing Corporation, 100 Avenue of the Americas, New York, New York, February 1992.

28. MacGregor, R.R. Alcohol and immune defense. *JAMA* 256 (11): pp. 1474-1479, 1986.

29. Gottesfeld, Z., and Abel, E.L. Minireview: Maternal and paternal alcohol use: Effects on the immune system of the offspring. *Life Sci* 48(1): pp. 1-8, 1991.

30. *Eighth Special Report to U.S. Congress on Alcohol and Health.* NIH Pub. No. 94-3699. Bethesada, MD: National Institutes of Health, op. cit., pp. xxi., 1993.

31. Kandel, D.B., and Andrews, K. Processes of adolescent socialization by parents and peers. *Int J Addict* 22(4): pp. 319-342, 1987.

32. Chaio YB, Van Thiel DH: Biochemical mechanisms that contribute to alcohol-induced hypogonadism in the male. *Alcoholism* (NY) 7(2): pp. 131-134, 1983.

33. Gavaler, J.S. Effects of moderate consumption of alcoholic beverages on endocrine function in post-menopausal women: Basis for hypothesis. In: Galanter, M., ed. *Recent Developments in Alcoholism.* Vol 6. New York: Plenum Press, 1988. pp. 229-251.

34. Zador, P.L. Alcohol-related relative risk of fatal driver injuries in relation to driver and age and sex. *J Stud Alcohol* 52(4): pp. 302-310, 1991.

Easy Order Form

HealthSpan Communications®

Please send: ***Shattering Myths & Mysteries of Alcohol***

➤ **Make check or money order payable to:**

HealthSpan Communications®
2726 Land Park Drive
Sacramento, CA 95818

❑ **Check enclosed**

❑ **Money order enclosed**

❑ VISA MasterCard **(Call HealthSpan) 916-443-2120**

Unit price per book:	**$14.95**
Sales tax per book: 7.75% for books shipped to **California** address.	**$1.16**
Shipping and handling per Book	**$2.39**

➤ **Total cost per book**

California	**$18.50**
Outside California	**$17.34**

➤ **Number of books** ______

➤ **Total payment enclosed** ______

➤ **Name** ______________________________

Company name ______________________________

Address ______________________________

City ____________________ **State** ______

Zip __________ **Date** ____________________

HealthSpan COMMUNICATIONS®

HealthSpan Communications' books, products, and seminars are designed to empower people, organizations, and businesses to enhance their level of well-being by providing insights and answers to common challenges.